# TIRED of being SICK and TIRED?

# TIRED of being SICK and TIRED?

## Wisdom for Health and Healing

Dr. Gilles Lamarche
Drs. Michel & Angel Dupuis
Dr. Randy Koski
Dr. D. J. LeDrew
Dr. Ernest Li
Dr. Don & Brandi MacDonald
Dr. James D. Powell
Dr. Nima Rahmany
Dr. Richard Tapper

INFINITE SOLUTIONS 4 YOU
TIMMINS, ONTARIO

www.InfiniteSolutions4You.com



The publisher recommends that readers discuss all actions with competent healthcare professionals before taking any action that may have been suggested in this book. While every effort has been made to ensure the accuracy of the material presented in this book, no warranties are provided as to the accuracy of information, and the publisher and co-authors cannot be held liable for errors or omissions pertaining to information contained herein. The opinions expressed are those of the individual authors and are not necessarily those of the other authors or of Infinite Solutions 4 You.

**Library and Archives Canada Cataloguing in Publication**

Tired of being sick and tired? : wisdom for health and healing / Gilles Lamarche ... [et al.].

ISBN 978-0-9782617-2-6

1. Chiropractic I. Lamarche, Gilles, 1955-

RZ241.T57 2008 615.5'34 C2008-902702-7

*Printed in Canada*

10 9 8 7 6 5 4 3 2 1

Cover and interior design by To The Point Solutions
www.tothepointsolutions.com

This book is dedicated to everyone who, throughout the ages, has contributed to sound health; to the professionals who endeavor to carry these messages forward; and to all people who benefit from this advice.

# Contents

# Preface

The most precious thing in life is your health. If you don't believe me, ask anyone who is chronically ill and/or fighting a disease what they want most, and they will tell you, without hesitation, "My health."

Have you ever wondered why people get sick? Why, for example, can a man live the first forty-five years of his life appearing completely healthy and then, all of a sudden, become extremely ill? Why does one virus cause only sniffles in one child but a serious disease in a sibling? Is it not logical to assume that if an individual is born healthy, with all systems functioning to their optimum, that this individual should, in fact, live a long healthy life? If science tells us that the human body is made to last 122 to 150 years, why is this not the case?

Society has come to recognize health as being "the absence of disease." Due to the quick-fix theory, people think that the answer to all ailments can be found in the utilization of a drug or chemical. Rather than looking for the *cause of health*, science has concentrated on trying to find the *cause of disease* and on defining the ability to fight disease.

It is strange that science appears to blame most illnesses on external forces, such as viruses and bacteria, because when we examine external forces, we find that one individual exposed to the exact same pathogen (disease-causing organism) will be seriously ill, while another person is unaffected. It has also been found that many individuals harbor serious pathogenic bacteria—while being completely asymptomatic.

Therefore, if we accept the theory that the primary cause of diseases are viruses and bacteria, how then do we explain the cause of various pathologies in which no virus or bacteria can be found?

We know that many paradigms exist concerning health and healing, some are similar to each other and some are not. Medicine and chiropractic, for example, are distinct and separate. Both professions have much to offer people who are sick. One is not inclusive of the other, and neither is exclusive.

Traditional medicine focuses on the disease and the avoidance of death. Chiropractic, on the other hand, focuses on health, the promotion of life, and searches for ways to free the nervous system to help restore health and vitality.

Traditional medicine works at curing a disease that has invaded an individual by utilizing chemical means or external invasive forces. It is mechanistic in nature, uses drugs to resist death, attempts to control the variables, battles the disease, and takes over the body's wisdom and works at relieving pain and postponing death. It cannot and does not restore health.

The wonderful advancements that have taken place regarding crisis-care are obvious; yet, at the same time, there have been major abuses of power. The fact that pharmaceutical companies want to control everything that is perceived as health or healthcare is definitely a concern.

The continued trend toward dependence on prescription and over-the-counter drugs is taking its toll on our health. This is something we can no longer afford to ignore, from a morbidity and mortality perspective, and also from a financial perspective. We spend more money per capita than ever before and yet the general health of our population is not improving.

The authors of the book *Squandering Billions—Health Care in Canada* tell a story that has existed for years, but has not been told before in such a blatant, unpretentious, and direct fashion. And the book *Death by Medicine*, authored by Gary Null, PhD; Carolyn Dean, MD, ND; Martin Feldman, MD; Debora Rosario, MD; and Dorothy Smith, PhD also points out that the crisis in healthcare is real.

According to the World Health Organization of the United Nations (WHO), Canada and the United States of America, which have great resources of scientific minds and technology, are statistically two of the unhealthiest countries in the developed world. Why is this?

Einstein said that you cannot solve a problem with the same level of thinking that created the problem in the first place. We must encourage all politicians, taxpayers, and health-care professionals to endorse the wisdom that is in this book.

*Tired of Being Sick and Tired?* is about bringing the truth to the surface and acknowledging that we can no longer expect to rule people with lies and deception. Dr. Pran Manga, PhD, a reputable and highly regarded epidemiologist from the University of Ottawa, has presented research to professionals and governments that could serve to improve the health of our communities and save taxpayers billions of dollars. Although extremely well respected among his peers, few of his ideas have been implemented.

My co-authors and I hope to change this.

# Introduction

You have healing power; we all do. If you want to improve your health and your life, read this book, which is sure to inspire you to new levels of awakening. As you read *Tired of Being Sick and Tired?*, you will be enlightened and your perspective on health and healing will be enhanced. You are certain to enjoy the thought-provoking and spine-chilling testimonials, as each author shares stories of what brought him or her to become a health-care professional. Find out what keeps them motivated to share their stories with you and others.

Some of the concepts in this book will challenge your beliefs and how you view previous life experiences. Remain open, devour the words, use multicolored highlighters to identify specific lessons, and keep this book nearby to review it often. By keeping it handy, you are sure to read a paragraph here and there to your friends in need. Perhaps you will request a second copy, so you can share it with those whom you love and for whom you want the absolute best health.

Healing is a science, a philosophy, and an art. It is duplicative, transferable, and, best of all, is available to you. By the end of this book, you will rewrite your own story of health and healing and give it a happier and more blissful ending.

Each contributing author is a colleague and a personal friend. Individually and collectively they live what they teach. They are competent professionals who exude confidence and perpetually go the extra mile to serve their patients and communities. Most importantly, all of them have imparted healing through their heads, hearts, hands—and now their words.

We collectively wish you a life that is inspiring and filled with health and well-being. We also ask that you give yourself permission to read and understand these words, and then awaken the healing power that lies within you.

Dr. Gilles Lamarche
Editor in Chief

"Many receive advice,
only the wise profit from it."

Syrus

TIRED of being
SICK and TIRED?

The five most dangerous words in the English language:

**Maybe it will go away.**

# 1.

# Is a Quick Fix Really the Answer?

## Dr. Gilles Lamarche, BSc, DC, DAc

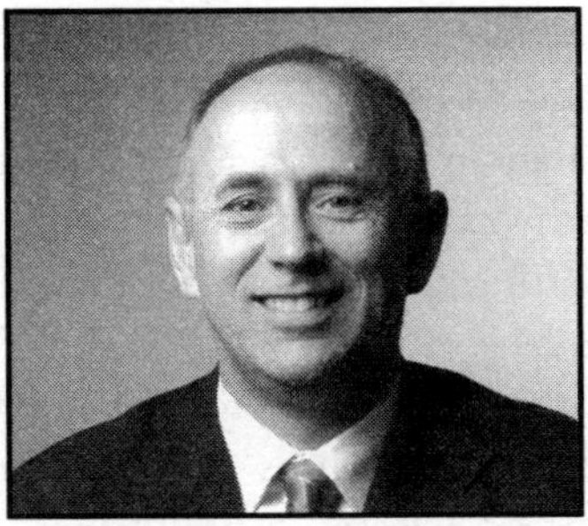

**Dr. Gilles Lamarche** was born and raised in Timmins, Ontario, Canada. At the age of twelve, he suffered from chronic back pain and was taken to a chiropractor. His only expectation was that a chiropractor might help him resume regular activities without pain. What he soon discovered, though, was a science and art that had as its main purpose the restoration of spinal function to enhance the health of the nervous system. This was a completely new paradigm for Lamarche, and a childhood of ill health soon became a thing of the past.

With improvement of his nervous-system health came improved digestion and bowel function. The signs and symptoms of *dis-ease* quickly disappeared and a vision developed: to help the world discover the importance and value of regular chiropractic care for overall health and well-being, a quest that he continues to live today, some forty-plus years later.

Lamarche attended the University of Toronto, graduating with a Bachelor of Science degree in 1975; and completed his postgraduate work at the Canadian Memorial Chiropractic College, receiving his Doctor of Chiropractic in 1979. He was in private practice in northern Ontario from 1979 to 2004, and is a recognized speaker on chiropractic (science, art, and philosophy), the art of healthy communication, and lifestyles for vibrant health.

In 2001, he was selected to appear in the National Registry's *Who's Who in Professionals and Executives, 2001-2002 Edition.*

In 2006, Dr. Lamarche was voted chiropractor of the year by his peers, the readers of *Canadian Chiropractor* magazine. The article that appeared in that magazine, written by Mr. David Stubbs, reveals many aspects of Dr. Lamarche's life and purpose. Stubbs writes: "With statistics showing that fewer than 12% of North Americans have utilized chiropractic, he is on a sort of 24/7 lecture tour that may find him explaining to a curious airport limousine driver what it is that chiropractors do. 'Why should chiropractic be a secret in healthcare?' he questions, and thus it has become his mission to better equip chiropractors to educate the public.

"From his perspective, it is in the public interest to make chiropractic accessible to all, an attitude he carries into his regulatory role as vice president of the executive committee of the Council of the College of Chiropractors of Ontario. Wearing yet another hat as a certified personal development coach, he can be found assisting practitioners through a series of exercises that help to clarify their sense of purpose, in the process revealing thinking patterns that are positive, as well as those that sabotage. 'It's all about the purpose you have for rendering the service you are rendering. Are you serving the person who is in front of you?' he asks."

During 2006 and 2007, Dr. Lamarche traveled more than 350,000 miles, speaking to audiences in Canada, the United

States, Australia, Japan, Mexico, Norway, England, and Scotland. He has received numerous awards for his commitment and dedication to helping mankind.

Dr. Lamarche has been involved with the College of Chiropractors of Ontario (CCO) as a member and chairman of the Patient Relations Committee, and in 1999 was elected to the Council of the CCO. He has chaired the Complaints Committee, has been vice president of the Executive Committee, and since 2006 has been president of the CCO.

For more than twenty years, Dr. Lamarche has been a featured speaker at the postgraduate seminars of the Parker College of Chiropractic and, in 2007, he became Director of Parker Seminars, the largest postgraduate chiropractic organization in the world.

A small man with a big heart, Dr. Lamarche's purpose statement reads: "I hereby pledge my life to my greatest expression of love and service for the benefit of humanity."

> "The doctor of the future will give no medicine, but will interest his patients in the care of the human frame, in diet, and in the cause in the prevention of disease."
>
> Thomas Edison

In a society where quick fixes are the request of the day, one wonders where and how this philosophy evolved. When drug commercials rule the media, one questions the service that is being provided, especially since chronic debilitating diseases continue to rise and alternative drugless health-care professions are ridiculed.

How long can we afford to let this health-care crisis fester before recognizing the agony it creates? Will we remain quiet and polite, or will we choose to stand up and utilize facts to win the battle of health and healthcare? When people are striving to discover health and wellness solutions, when statistics show that people are willing to pay out-of-pocket for true healthcare, will politicians listen or will we continue to experience more technology and debt, and less health?

> "Understand you but waste time, unless you go beyond what you have learned to what is yet to learn."
> A Gift of Peace/Course in Miracles

This is not a fictional story; it is a compilation of truths. The references and facts in this chapter leave little to the imagination. When you read this information and realize what we have allowed to transpire, you are likely to have a sick feeling of dissolution. Our present health-care system is like a freight train moving forward at a very high speed with little or no checks and balances to stop it.

This is a trend we cannot ignore any longer.

On April 22, 2005, *New York Times* columnist Paul Krugman wrote: "Americans spend more on healthcare than anyone else . . . Yet we have the highest infant mortality and close to the lowest life expectancy of any wealthy nation."

Why has the system focused almost solely on crisis intervention when, in fact, research often describes the importance of health-care choices that encourage proactive approaches? Here are some of the facts and answers.

Prescription drugs constitute the major treatment modality of today's so-called scientific medicine. It is an outside-in approach that is based on the germ theory: that infectious organisms are the cause of illness.

Finding the cure for infections proved harder than anyone imagined and, over the years, research has shown that many bacteria that would cause disease if they were in one part of your body are actually a healthy aspect of other systems in your body. For instance, it is normal to have certain bacteria in your bowel, but if the same bacteria were in your mouth or outside your intestines they would, in fact, be deadly to you.

Thus, in their quest to fight these organisms, scientists invented numerous chemical drugs—and they have delivered much less than promised. As a matter of fact, most of these drugs, when prescribed and utilized as directed, cause incalculable side effects that can be fatal. According to Jason Lazarou, MSc: "Human error or improper prescription can make the situation even worse. In a *New England Journal of Medicine* study, one in four patients suffered observable side effects from the more than 3.34 billion drug prescriptions filled in 2002."[1]

> "Always remember that good health is a natural state. Years ago people did not die of lifestyle diseases. They died of old age or trauma. Your health is your responsibility. Learn to make good choices."
>
> Dr. Gilles Lamarche

William Tierney, editor of this study said, "Given the increasing number of powerful drugs available to care for the aging population, the problem will only get worse."[2] Apparently over 5 percent of hospital admissions (over 1 million per year) are the result of drug side effects. This number does not take into account the amount of drug reactions that occur to patients while they are in the hospital.[3] Furthermore, most of these reactions are never documented or reported.

> "The quality of your life is dependent on the quality of the questions you are willing to ask. What questions are you asking concerning your life?"
>
> Les Brown

Prescription and over-the-counter drugs are available for any symptom or condition, most of which could be rectified with lifestyle and behavior changes. People who seek more enjoyment and relief from stress become prey for the TV advertisements that suggest drugs are the answer.

We fight the illegal street drug trade, yet allow pharmaceutical companies to market so-called legal drugs (because they are supposed to be regulated), and forget about the serious damage these drugs cause the people who use them and society as a whole.

An entire generation of antidepressant users has been created by young people growing up on Ritalin because parents and teachers alike refused to face up to the fact that different children learn differently; that over-stimulation can lead to inattention; and that, in fact, children need love and attention rather than more video games.

There is a real need to go back to traditional family values as part of creating healthy beings and healthy societies.

Medicating people and modifying their emotions has an impact on how they learn to deal with their feelings. People cope by using drugs rather than discovering what lies within. As adults, these "medicated youth" no doubt reach for other substances, whether considered legal or illegal. According to the *Journal of the American Medical Association (JAMA)*, the commonly prescribed youth drug Ritalin acts much like cocaine.[4]

The marketing of drugs, such as Prozac and Zoloft, makes them not only socially acceptable; people think it weird if you are not using any. Years ago, pharmaceutical companies marketed directly to physicians. Watch any television channel today and you will view multiple ads suggesting that you, the viewer, ask your physician about a certain drug.

Yes, companies are marketing directly to the consumer and creating demand at the grassroots level. By 1995, drug companies had tripled the amount of money allotted to direct advertising of prescription drugs to consumers. The majority of this money is spent on seductive television ads. From 1996 to 2000, spending rose from $791 million to $2.5 billion.[5] This $2.5 billion represents only 15 percent of the total pharmaceutical advertising budget. Do the calculation. If $2.5 billion is 15 percent, the total spent on advertising drugs is $16.6 billion.

Viewers are often misinformed about these drugs. One important study found that people mistakenly believe that the Federal Drug Administration (FDA) reviews all ads before they are released and allows only the safest and most effective drugs to be promoted.[6] Drugs are usually tested on individuals who are healthy and not taking other medications that could affect the findings of the study. Once the drugs are declared safe and enter the prescription book library, they are prescribed to people who may be using a variety of different drugs and who are ill. The effects are sometimes devastating.

This reminds me of my grandmother. When she was in her mid-seventies, she became very ill and depressed. Upon taking her to a cardiologist, who took appropriate time to consult with her and conduct the necessary testing, it was declared that my grandmother's symptoms were all effects of the drugs her family physician had prescribed. The cardiologist systematically weaned my grandmother off these drugs and my grandmother lived until the age of ninety-four.

So much is unknown about drugs and their effects. Although drugs are put through a pre-approval process, they are also supposed to go through a post-approval process that requires proper reporting and documentation of any side effects. In one important report, the U.S. government's General Accounting Office "found that of the 198 drugs approved by the FDA between 1976 and 1985 . . . 102 (or 51%) had serious post-approval risks . . . the serious post-approval risks (included) heart failure, myocardial infarction, anaphylaxis, respiratory depression and arrest, seizures, kidney and liver failure, severe blood disorders, birth defects and fetal toxicity, and blindness."[7]

Other studies show consistent misuse of medications, such as antibiotics. Almost half the patients with upper respiratory tract infections in the U.S. still receive antibiotics from their doctors,[8] when according to the Center for Disease Control (CDC), 90% of upper respiratory infections are viral in nature, do not respond to antibiotics, and should not be treated with antibiotics.

Data in the U.S. indicates that on average, every child receives 1.22 antibiotic prescriptions annually. I had the honor and privilege of fathering three children, who today are twenty-five, twenty-four, and twenty-two years old. Not one of them ever received an antibiotic, needle, lotion, or potion—as would normally be prescribed as "necessary" by traditional medicine. To this day, they are healthy.

And, their good health is the result of a drug-free chiropractic lifestyle, which you will learn much about in this book, and of healthy lifestyle choices and a nervous system free of interference.

Deficiency + Toxicity = Disease
Sufficiency + Purity = Health
Are you getting sufficient rest, quality food and water, and nervous system transmission? Are you creating a balanced life where you take time for play, work, and exercise? Do you feed your mind positive, healthy thoughts? Do you choose love and gratitude? If not, what different choices will you start making—today?

Dr. Gilles Lamarche

In *Death by Medicine,* the authors provide statistics from a variety of studies published in reputable medical and scientific journals. These statistics are revealing and are sure to awaken you.

- Each year approximately 2.2 million U.S. hospital patients experience adverse drug reactions (ADRs) to prescribed medications.[9] In 1995, Dr. Richard Besser of the CDC estimated the number of unnecessary antibiotics prescribed annually for viral infections to be 20 million; in 2003, Dr. Besser spoke in terms of tens of millions of unnecessary antibiotics prescribed annually.*10* Approximately 7.5 million unnecessary medical and surgical procedures are performed annually in the U.S.,[11] while approximately 8.9 million Americans are hospitalized unnecessarily.[12]

- Deaths inadvertently induced by a physician or surgeon or medical treatment or diagnostic procedure in the U.S. annually equal 783,936. It is evident that the American medical system is the leading cause of death and injury in that country. By comparison, approximately 699,697 Americans died of heart disease in 2001, and 553,251 died of cancer.[13] According to other researchers utilizing postulates by Leape[14], the number of deaths caused by medicine would be closer to 999,936.
- The estimated ten-year total of deaths by medicine is more than all the casualties from all the wars fought by the U.S. throughout its history. (If that number does not shock you and entice you to look at alternatives for your health and well-being, nothing will.)

> "Ninety percent of our behaviors are habitual. Your habits are only getting you what you are currently getting. If you want something different, you must choose to think differently and develop new habits."
>
> Jack Canfield

According to an ABC News report, pharmaceutical companies spend more than $2 billion annually on over 314,000 events attended by physicians. The ABC news report also noted that a survey of clinical trials revealed that when a drug company funds a study, there is a 90 percent chance that the drug will be perceived as affective whereas a non-drug-company-funded study will show favorable results only 50 percent of the time. They concluded by saying it appears that money can't buy you love but it can buy you any "scientific" result desired.

Rudy Giuliani, the former mayor of New York City and short-term GOP candidate for U.S. president, has said that "the cost of medical care in the United States exceeds two trillion dollars annually, and costs are continuing to rise. Policy makers must consider strategies to make healthcare more affordable and portable without compromising the quality of care. There is a growing body of evidence that services provided by doctors of chiropractic reduce health-care costs, improve health behaviors, and enhance patient quality of life. The results of several patient-based studies suggest that chiropractic care may result in significant savings of health-care dollars. The federal government has recognized chiropractic services as an appropriate form of healthcare. Chiropractic services have been covered under the Medicare program since 1972.

"More recently, legislation has been enacted that provides for chiropractic services in the Department of Defense and the Veteran's Administration. Doctors of Chiropractic have proven to be important assets to our communities. As president, I will defend your rights to practice your trade. I will support the freedom of American citizens to choose chiropractic healthcare and to have access to chiropractic services to improve their health and quality of life."

When politicians start to acknowledge the value in chiropractic care, there is hope that methods that can help you discover and maintain your health may, in time, become mainstream.

Dr. Carlon Colker, an internal medicine physician from Connecticut, and one of the world's foremost experts in optimizing health and performance, released two CDs in 2007—*The Cure Conspiracy: Why Some Doctors Won't Lie* and *The Cure Conspiracy: Why My Partner is a Chiropractor.*[15] He reveals important information as to why and how our health system is near collapse and urges us to look at alternate methods to discover and maintain our health. Some of the most poignant facts he relates are:

- The very industry that was created to help us be healthy actually doesn't make cures at all; it actually has a vested financial interest in keeping us sick.
- Drug companies manufacture drugs that create a dependency so you will need them forever.
- Drugs just manage your symptoms. They do not cure anything.
- Physicians are taught that the only things to help people be healthy are drugs and surgery.
- Physicians should be skeptical of anything outside of that paradigm. Words like *alternative, integrated, herbal, nutrition, naturopath, chiropractic, nature* or anything not entrenched in the medical system should conjure up images of witch doctors and are, by nature, bad.
- Physicians are taught that if it is not an FDA-approved drug or procedure, they should automatically reject and stay away from it. On this basis alone, drug com-

panies and the FDA say that drugs are cures and nature is the alternative.

- The fact is that nature holds the cure, and it is drugs that are the alternative.
- The FDA will not allow statements regarding the treatment or cure of any disease to be applied to natural supplements. According to the FDA, only a drug that they have been paid by "Big Pharma" to approve can be said to treat or cure a disease.
- Making wise decisions for your health and to prevent diseases is the essence of wellness.
- The most common diseases, such as coronary artery disease, high blood pressure, and diabetes, are managed by drugs that do not cure or reverse the disease process. None of the countless drugs on the market cure these diseases; what they do is manage the signs and symptoms of the disease. They do not address why the person got sick in the first place.
- The medical system believes that only a drug that the FDA has been paid to approve holds the cures.
- Dr. Colker prides himself on avoiding drugs at all costs, whenever possible. He believes that drugs actually pollute the body's internal environment. Drugs should be used only when you are left with no other option.
- A patient's illness should not just be matched to a corresponding drug while paying no attention to what else could be done to improve health and avoid the drug altogether.

- Nearly every drug has a laundry list of potential side effects, many of which are deadly.
- Supplements and natural remedies actually hold the answer to many cures, but drugs do not. Nature is critically important to the maintenance of a healthy individual.
- We may be more health conscious, but we are not necessarily healthier. Our present generation is the first generation that is expected to have a shorter lifespan than its parents.
- At one point Americans were the tallest people; now they are one of the shortest and fattest. Obesity and obesity-related illnesses are at an all-time high.
- The National Cancer Institute admitted that between 1973 and 1993 the incidence of cancer and cancer-related deaths escalated.
- Even with the advent of no-fat and low-fat foods, heart disease is still the number one killer disease.
- Despite doctors prescribing more drugs than ever, diseases such as asthma, cancer, diabetes, and heart disease are at an all-time high.
- We are in the middle of a health-care hurricane, a true calamity. And we are missing the cures, which are right under our noses.
- The major malfunction is how we approach health in the first place. Society has this notion that if you are not sick your body does not need attention. This is the obvious way of missing a solution. We must maintain our health just like we maintain our cars and homes.

- Dietary supplements and what is offered by chiropractors are health-based. Physicians offer disease care, not healthcare. Physicians actually lack the information to help you get well and stay well naturally, because they are trained to prescribe drugs.
- You can optimize your health. Do not let closed-minded doctors and drug companies govern your thinking about health and healing.
- Nature is more powerful than any drug, which is why drug companies lobby so strongly against anything natural a body needs to be healthy. Natural remedies have great value, especially when used as prevention.
- People have been convinced they must take medications rather than make wise decisions to focus on prevention and take responsibility for their lifestyles.
- Drug companies are exploiting the senior population by making them believe they need multiple drugs for survival when, in fact, this is making many seniors even sicker.
- Our health is priceless and drug companies exploit this natural want by charging premium amounts. We can no longer pay this ransom.
- One of the greatest destructors of health is the release of free radicals that create disease at the cellular/molecular level.
- The body is designed to gravitate towards wellness and heal itself. Real health comes from nature. Everything you need to heal yourself is found within you and in nature.

- The primary cause of disease is the oxidation process, which can best be described as rusting. To avoid the damages of oxidation, it is important to choose foods and supplements that are high in their anti-oxidation activities. At the top of the list is the acai fruit.
- Modern medicine is starting to recognize the value of diet as it relates to health and well-being.
- Natural cures are available. Visit a health-care practitioner who understands this.
- Disease prevention is the key. Do what you can to prevent disease and get involved in a prevention program that is supported by your health-care practitioner.

Dr. Colker's call to action is to look at natural methods that will help you live better and stronger. For years, chiropractors have promoted the belief that nature cures and your body has the ability to heal itself, provided there is no interference. A chiropractor is your ideal partner to discovering and maintaining great health.

Health is not found in a pill or a potion. Good health truly comes from within and is available to you. You must first believe that health is there for you and start making the right choices to experience this wonderful gift.

> "Every day, commit to doing one thing that you know will make you happy and healthy."
> Jack Canfield

Yes, health is a choice and is dependent on you consistently making the right choices day in and day out. It starts with the belief that health is available to you.

Many think that the benefits and seemingly miraculous

results of belief are based on speculative or abstract reasoning, or the metaphysical. However, this is not the case. The power of belief is proven almost daily in the scientific community and is known as the placebo effect. Do you believe that you can be healthy and experience the life that you aspire to live?

When researchers test the effectiveness of new drugs on humans, they give the drug to some of the volunteers and they give a *placebo*, or an inactive substance or preparation, to the others. In almost all cases, some of the volunteers that were given the placebo report the same effects as those who were given the actual drug.

Irving Kirsch, a psychologist at the University of Connecticut, believes that the effectiveness of Prozac and similar drugs may be attributed almost entirely to the placebo effect. He and Guy Sapirstein analyzed nineteen clinical trials of antidepressants and concluded that the expectation of improvement, not adjustments in brain chemistry, accounted for 75 percent of the drugs' effectiveness (Kirsch 1998). "The critical factor," says Kirsch, "is our belief about what's going to happen to us. You don't have to rely on drugs to see profound transformation."[16]

> "Success, health, and happiness are often not about adding anything, but a shedding process; a process where you eliminate what is creating distress to both mind and body."
>
> Dr. James W. Parker

Dr. Deepak Chopra, best-selling author and one of the leaders in the field of mind, body, and spirit healing, is an advocate of the power of belief and its seemingly miraculous effects on the body. He cites several studies of patients with multiple personality disorder who display different physical traits with each personality, like visible allergic reactions on the skin, high blood pressure, and even different eye color. He also discusses cases where several of his patients have used the power of belief to get rid of cancer in their bodies.

Success is having belief and not going though life as a cynical skeptic. Remember, thought and imagination are limitless. The body and spirit often are limited by what one believes is possible.

Prior to Roger Bannister breaking the four-minute barrier to running one mile in 1954, no one else was able to achieve this goal and many thought it was not humanly possible. Shortly after Bannister's new record, other runners broke the self-imposed mental barrier and broke the four-minute mile as well.

There is a metaphysical part to belief. This theory states that when you truly believe in something, the forces of the universe work toward making that belief a manifestation, or giving physical form to the belief. A great example of this is health.

Believe you will succeed and you will. Believe in your own abilities and have faith in yourself. As Napoleon Hill, one of the early-twentieth-century experts in success wrote:

> "Whatever the human mind can conceive and believe, it can achieve."

The content of this book will challenge some of your beliefs about health and healing. You will find yourself questioning what you have learned about health from your environment—family and friends, physicians, school teachers, and others.

The health-care system in North America is in serious trouble. We spend more money per capita than all other countries, and yet the residents of Canada and the U.S. are not the healthiest people in the world. We have become the product of commercialized propaganda and have made many decisions about health that actually lead to increased disease and morbidity.

Read this book with an open mind and remember what Albert Einstein said: "You cannot solve a problem with the same level of thinking that created the problem in the first place."

To achieve better results with your health, you must be willing to think differently, look at the options available, and make wiser decisions.

For more information or to book Dr. Lamarche as a speaker at your next health and wellness event, visit his website at:

www.gilleslamarche.com

## Chapter Notes

1. Lazarou, Jason MsC; Bruce H. Pomeranz, MD, PhD; and Paul N. Corey, PhD. "Incidence of Adverse Drug Reactions in Hospitalized Patients: A Meta-Analysis of Prospective Studies," *JAMA*. April 15, 1998: 279(15); 1200-5.

2. Foster, AJ, Murff HJ, Peterson JF, Gandhi TK, Bates DW. "The incidence and severity of adverse events affecting patients after discharge from hospital." *Annals of Internal Medicine*, 2003 Feb 4; 138(3):161-7.

3. Medication side effects strike 1 in 4. Reuters. April 17, 2003.

4. Vastag B. "Pay Attention: Ritalin acts much like cocaine." *JAMA*. 2001 August 22-29; 286(8):905-6.

5. Wolfe, SM. Direct to consumer advertising—education or emotion promotion? *New England Journal of Medicine*. 2002 February 14;346(7):524-6.

6. Ibid.

7. Agger, WA. Antibiotics resistance: unnatural selection in the office and on the farm. *Wisconsin Medical Journal*, August 2002.

8. Rabin, R. Caution about overuse of antibiotics. *Newsday*, September 18, 2003. 8a. Centers for Disease Control and Prevention. CDC antimicrobial resistance and antibiotic resistance-general information. Available at http://www.cdc.gov/drugresistance/community/. As on December 13, 2003.

9. Lazarou, Jason MsC; Bruce H. Pomeranz, MD, PhD; and Paul N. Corey, PhD. "Incidence of Adverse Drug Reactions in Hospitalized Patients: A Meta-Analysis of Prospective Studies," *JAMA*. April 15, 1998: 279(15); 1200-5.

10. See note 8.

11. Unnecessary Surgery. Sources: HCUPnet, Healthcare Cost and Utilization Project. Agency for Healthcare Research and Quality, Rockville,Maryland. Available at http://www.ahrq.gov/data/hcup/hcupnet.html

12. Unnecessary Hospitalizations. Available at http://www.ahrq.gov/data/hcup/hcupnet.htm

13. U.S. National Center for Health Statistics. *National Vital Statistics Report*, vol.51 no.5, March 14, 2003.

14. Nationwide poll on patient safety: 100 million Americans see medical mistakes directly touching them [press release]. McLean, VA : National Patient Safety Foundation; October 9, 1997.

15. http://www.cureconspiracy.com

16. Kirsch, Irving, PhD and Sapirstein, Guy, PhD, "Listening to Prozac but Hearing Placebo: A Meta Analysis of Antidepressant Medication," *Prevention and Treatment*, Volume 1, June 1998.

# 2.

# THE KITCHEN SINK THEORY

## DR. DON AND BRANDI MACDONALD

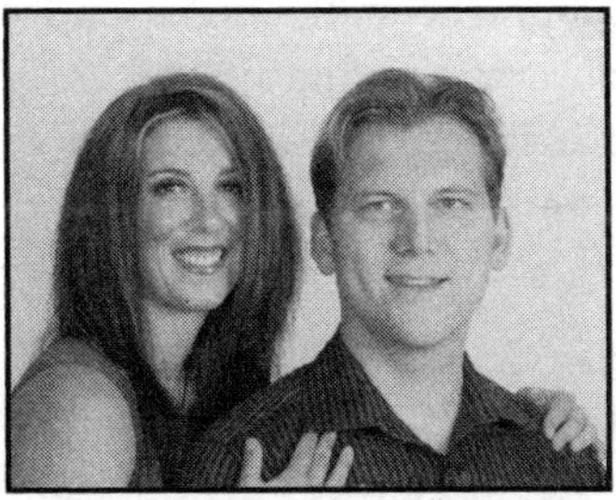

**Dr. Don MacDonald** was inspired to become a chiropractor after chiropractic helped him with chronic knee tendonitis and asthma. In 1997, he graduated from Palmer College of Chiropractic. Since then he has owned and actively practiced in a busy clinic in Edmonton, Alberta. Dr. Don is President of the Edmonton Chiropractic Society and is a member of the Marketing Committee for the Alberta Chiropractic College and Association. His mission is to help change people's perception of health from a sick-care model to a wellness-proactive model. Dr. Don can be reached at www.whitemudcrossingchiropractors.com or by phone at 780-430-7549.

For over ten years, **Brandi MacDonald** led large multi-disciplinary teams that supported women, children, and families living in poverty. By the time she was twenty-seven, she was promoted to the position of Executive Director. After ten years of working in the non-profit industry, she decided to open up her own business. She was later touched by the healing power of chiropractic and left her successful career to spread the message of chiropractic and inspirational leadership. Brandi is a patient of chiropractic, an advocate of wellness, wife of a chiropractor, and a motivating leader.

Currently, she manages a multi-doctor, high-volume clinic for her husband, Dr. Don MacDonald. She is the owner of True Concepts Inc., which consults with chiropractors on how to hire, retain, and inspire staff. She travels across Canada and the United States to train chiropractic staff on the philosophy and art of being a chiropractic assistant. She also provides leadership training to chiropractors. Brandi can be reached at www.brandimacdonald.com or by e-mail at bj.mac@shaw.ca.

## Everything you need to know about health is in your kitchen sink.

Usually when patients come into a chiropractic office they have tried everything else and are frustrated that they have not been able to regain their health. This is a perfect opportunity for them to learn how the body works and I like to use the analogy of a kitchen sink to teach them how they can look after themselves better.

Chiropractic is powerful on its own, but when people understand why the human body responds the way it does, it gives them an advantage on their road to recovery and they can then move forward toward living healthy and fulfilling lives.

What does a kitchen sink have to do with getting and staying healthy? Let me explain.

Imagine a kitchen, including the sink, stove, and fridge. The floor has just been redone with the most expensive, immaculate hardwood. You are very proud of this new floor. And, in order to keep it in great shape, no water can be spilled on it.

Now, let's say that this nicely finished floor represents your overall health. If the sink, which represents the body and nervous system, overflows, water will spill onto the hardwood causing it to deteriorate, and eventually destroy it. The same thing happens to your body when excess stress builds up. If the stress becomes more than what your body and nervous system can handle, things go wrong and you start to lose your health.

Sinks come in various sizes. Yours may be small and able to hold a little water, or large and able to hold a lot before it overflows and ruins the floor (or in this case, your health).

To preclude your sink from overflowing, there are some preventive measures you can take. One is to be sure you are not adding water faster than the drain can release it. Another is to ensure that the drain has no clogs or obstructions.

A kitchen sink has a tap and a drain. The tap brings water into the sink or, in this analogy, stress flows into your daily life as an unavoidable aspect of living. (We will divide this stress into four different types later.) A rule I am going to throw into the mix is that the tap cannot be turned off. Water will flow continuously into the sink, just as the stress of living constantly invades your body and nervous system.

In this image, the drain represents stress relief: the method the body and nervous system use to release the buildup of stress and keep the life force flowing without permanent damage to your health.

If there is a lack of stress releasers, stress will accumulate in your body. If nothing is changed, these stressors will ruin your health.

By the end of this chapter you will know five strategies to decrease your stress and increase your stress releasers so you can apply them in your daily life to regain your health and to proactively live a wellness lifestyle.

## The water pouring from the tap represents the stress in your life.

The tap water that fills the sink is similar to the stressors you accumulate by having a full life. Basically, there are four types of stress: Physical, Emotional, Chemical, and Electromagnetic. These are the causes of what chiropractors call *subluxation* or *misalignment of the spine,* which create abnormal movement and nerve interference.

1. **Physical Stress** is caused by different activities you engage in. Many patients do not realize what damage has been accumulating. Some work on computers and compromise their postures daily as they peer at the screen. Others have physical jobs that demand heavy lifting and/or repetitive movement. Physical stress can also be caused by car accidents, sports injuries, childhood falls, sleeping incorrectly, bad posture habits, etc. Many people think that physical stress is the only cause of subluxations, but in clinical practice, we find that emotional stress is the main culprit.

2. **Emotional Stress** is caused by fear, guilt, anger, resentment, excitement, sadness, frustration, worry, and any other emotion that keeps your mind continuously active. The problem with emotional stress is that it is

difficult to eliminate or lessen. It is much easier to tell a patient to lift correctly or to make sure their work station is ergonomically correct than it is to tell them to stop worrying about family, work, or financial problems.

Emotional stress is the number one reason people lose their health. Basically, your tap is on full blast, thus creating a huge problem if you are not keeping the drain clear and open. Emotional stress is pervasive. One of the best ways we have discovered to dissolve emotions is by following Dr. John Demartini's advice. A fellow chiropractor and one of the speakers on the bestselling DVD, *The Secret,* he has developed the Demartini Method to collapse emotional charges. You can find resources on how to alleviate stress on his website: www.drdemartini.com.

3. **Chemical Stress** is caused by any substance that is toxic to your internal environment. This can include air and water pollution, chemicals in food, and recreational and prescription drugs. Whenever your body has to break down a toxic substance, your nervous system goes into a fight-or-flight response, which adds to your stress levels.

   The environment we live in today is much different than it was one generation ago. We now have poorer quality of food, air, and water. Oftentimes you don't even know what new chemicals you are being exposed to, so it is difficult to control. But, by limiting the chemicals you know to be hazardous to your health, you will go a long way to protecting yourself and enhancing your wellness.

4. **Electromagnetic Stress** is a relatively new phenomenon. With the invention of electrical devices, humans are now bombarded with electromagnetic stress. Whenever an electric device is used it gives off an electromagnetic field—and it is rare if anyone goes one day without being exposed to this stress. To alleviate this influence, we recommend that you avoid sleeping on a heated water bed or utilizing an electric blanket. Also, keep your electric alarm clock away from the bed so you are not exposed while you sleep.

The amount of stress the human body can safely handle is limited. When stress accumulates excessively, the brain helps by turning down the body's awareness. This can be experienced as an increase in pain tolerance or a decrease in sensation. These, however, are short-term fixes because the brain and body must be tuned in with one other in order to effectively communicate and to respond appropriately.

Many of our patients have been under so much stress they say they feel like they are not in their bodies. They feel spaced out and have a hard time concentrating. This is one reason why it is important to both decrease the stress in your life and learn how to relax.

## The drain represents stress releasers in your life.

You know it is important not to allow the kitchen sink to overflow, as it will ruin the new hardwood floor. For the drain to be kept free of any buildup, restriction, or blockage you must be vigilant at employing a variety of methods such as cleaners, wire snakes, and drain plungers.

Likewise, there are five ways you can help release the stress in your body: having a proper nerve supply, exercise, sufficient rest, good nutrition, and living a life of purpose. The more you work on these five stress releasers the more water you are going to drain from the sink and prevent it from overflowing.

1. Proper nerve supply is a result of the spine being in alignment and functioning properly. Two of the first things to develop in a fetus are the brain and spinal cord. Developing next are the nerves that branch out from the spinal cord, and then all else develops around this. When the spinal nerves that regulate growth become irritated, the body and brain have difficulty communicating with each other. This intercommunication between body and mind needs to be both efficient and immediate. If the body and brain are not working together for self-regulation and adaptation, the body will begin to deteriorate.

   As chiropractors, we call this condition a *subluxation*. Subluxation is the malfunction of a spinal joint that interferes with nerve supply. You have twenty-four bones in your spine that create joints with each other. Between each joint is a small opening that allows the spinal nerve to exit from the spinal cord to the rest of the body. Any pressure on these nerves or a malfunction of the spinal joint results in subluxation.

   Many diseases that we know of today can be linked back to stress accumulation. A great test to tell if you might have spinal subluxations is to check your posture. Poor posture puts extra stress on the spine, thus increasing your chances of subluxation. The best way to determine if you have nerve interference is to be evaluated by a chiropractor. Chiropractic is the only profession that is trained to detect and correct spinal subluxations for the purpose of allowing the body's inborn ability to heal itself. It doesn't matter what problems you are having, if you address them early it takes much less time, energy, and money to correct them. It is always better to be proactive than reactive.

2. Exercise is essential to staying healthy. Stress has a way of building up in muscles as tension. Tension will not usually release with only your will to do so. Muscles need activity and movement to release and relax tension. Activities as simple as going for a walk, a swim, or a yoga session will enable the muscles to ease off.

   There are pros and cons involved in exercise. Yes, exercise is valuable to create a relaxation response and turn off the stress response, but exercise can also cause problems if done improperly. The main goal is to burn off excess stress and energy without hurting yourself.

   Excessive exercise can cause problems, so moderation and proper form are key. If you have never worked-out before, consult your chiropractor, wellness coach, or a certified personal trainer to learn how to get yourself in tiptop shape. Many people have improved their health immensely by training—and unfortunately, some have also been hurt in the process. If you injure yourself, you can set yourself back weeks or months in the healing process. If you experience such a setback, it will be less likely you will continue to exercise in the long run, and that would not be helpful to your long-term health and well-being. Respect and honor your body by starting any exercise program gradually and build up slowly. You will definitely see the results. Like all good things, exercise results take time.

3. Since the invention of the light bulb, lack of sleep has become a chronic problem for many people.

Televisions, computers, and other electrical devices serve as distracters and entice you to stay awake into the early hours of the morning. With the hectic pace most people live, the body needs more time to rebuild and relax. There are also other reasons why adequate sleep is often outside our grasp, such as stress, tension in the body, or an overactive brain.

Even if you spend eight or nine hours in bed, you can rise in the morning feeling exhausted if you fail to get into a deep sleep. Realize, these stress releasers work together. If you start with chiropractic care, you will relieve the stress on the nervous system, which will help you get a good night's sleep. If you begin regular exercise, your muscles will be more likely to relax and relieve nervous system tension, enabling you to sleep better.

4. Good nutrition is essential for stress release and repair. When a body is trying to rebuild itself, it needs good materials. Your cells are continuously being renewed. What raw materials are you providing for this re-construction? You can build two kitchens using the exact same blueprints, but one kitchen is built with top-grade materials and the other is built with scraps from the dump. Which will be of better quality? Which is likely to perform optimally? Of course, the one built with the top-of-the-line materials is more apt to perform better.

   The North American diet has fallen to its lowest quality since the history of the human race. For the most part, people eat highly processed foods that lack nutrients and are high in sugar, plus they ingest pesticides from many fruits and vegetables. This poor diet, in combination with lack of exercise and high levels of stress, creates problems such as heart disease and cancer—the leading causes of preventable death. With a high-paced lifestyle and fast-food restaurants on every corner, it takes discipline and planning on your part to be certain to get the nutrients your body needs to thrive, relax, repair, and rebuild.

5. The last stress releaser is to create a purposeful life for yourself. Many people work fulltime and function in a constant state of obligation. How many times have you heard someone say, "I only have x amount of years to go before I can retire and leave this crazy job"? Most people who utilize such expressions go through the same cycle week after week for years: "Monday blues," then "hump day Wednesday," and finally "thank God it's Friday." Saturday they rest because of the hard week and then on Sunday they begin to get anxious because tomorrow they have to go back to work. They simply go through the motions while waiting for something better.

   Finding joy in what you do is a therapeutic process and necessary if you want to have a life that is pleasurable. People who enjoy what they do and find ways to benefit others are healthier and live longer.

   Those who live by obligation typically enter retirement without a plan or any hobbies. Research has shown that most retirees end up dying within several months or a couple of years at most after retiring because they have lost their purpose in life. This is ironic since most people look forward to the day they can retire.

   With planning, you can find a way to serve others, and

> then your life will be a blessing rather than a drudgery, whether you are retired or not.
>
> Like the other four stress releasers, this is an area to research and learn about. Realize the more that you put these methods of relaxation into practice, the more peace, health, and happiness you will experience.

Now that you have several ways to keep stress down and your health up, analyze the stressors in your life and make a list of everything that you are exposed to in the four areas of stress. Spend a few days doing this to make sure you have all of the stressors written down.

Once you have a complete list, read through it and see which stressors would be easiest to lessen or eliminate completely. Sometimes you expose yourself to stressful things or situations just because you always have. Awareness is the key. If you are going through life on autopilot you may not realize how you are treating yourself and your body. If you are having a hard time decreasing your stress, get help from someone or hire a coach.

To get more information on alleviating stress, visit our website and sign up for our "Empty Your Kitchen Sink" newsletter at www.howisyoursink.com. This newsletter will help you discover ways to make sure you do not let your kitchen sink overflow.

After you have reduced the stressors in your life, it is time to start increasing your stress releasers. The strategy for this is to write down the five stress releasers discussed earlier and make a list under each one, choosing one or two things you can add or detract from your life that would keep the stress down.

You can start with a small change in your diet, like drinking more water and cutting down on sweets. You may want to start walking for ten to fifteen minutes each night or go to bed thirty minutes earlier every evening. You can go to a chiropractor and get a full spinal and nervous system examination to see if you have subluxations. And, you can start a journey toward discovering your talents and what you would love to bring to the world to make it a better place.

Remember, by making small changes and adding a few good habits and taking away a few negative ones, your body will start to function better and you will start to heal.

Below are our personal life stories that explain how chiropractic and the kitchen sink technique helped change our lives.

## How I Became a Chiropractor

Dr. Don MacDonald

In high school, I fell in love with basketball. I had a one-track mind. Everything I did was focused on shooting hoops, including researching workout programs, working out longer to become stronger, and practicing my shots.

I participated in a few summer basketball camps and started to see myself improve as a player. In eleventh grade, though, my knees started to hurt as soon as I got up in the morning and especially after running and jumping. I began to get concerned because the pain was affecting my ability to play. I was not as quick and couldn't jump as high.

My medical doctor diagnosed me with jumper's knee. He prescribed anti-inflammatory drugs, which I took on a regular basis, along with painkillers. About this time, I asked my parents if I could move into the city for my senior year, to live with my aunt and uncle, which would allow me to play in a more competitive basketball league. My parents were supportive, so I moved to the city.

With increased competition came increased practices. I was playing five to six times per week and my condition deteriorated rapidly. At seventeen I had a hard time running without wearing knee braces. I was taking painkillers and icing my knees before and after practices and games. A physiotherapist told me that one part of my anterior thigh muscle was over developed, so they administered ultrasound and muscle stimulation. I studied about leg muscles and tried to correct this muscle imbalance in my workouts. I then noticed my breathing became labored whenever I played. My coach insisted on extra conditioning because he thought I was out of shape. Another medical doctor diagnosed my labored breathing as exercise-induced asthma.

I went off to college to play basketball; but continued to struggle with knee pain and the asthma.

It was at this point my sister attended a career day at her school. She wanted to be either a medical doctor or a physiotherapist so she listened to both presentations. She was allowed a third speaker, so she attended the chiropractor's talk. After listening to the three speakers, she decided on the spot to become a chiropractor. She heard Dr. Duane Smethurst talk about how the body had an inborn ability to heal itself, that it was controlled by the nervous system, and if there was interference to that system, the body would not function at its optimal potential.

She asked Dr. Duane if he would be able to help her brother's knees and breathing. He replied that he wouldn't know for sure until after he had given me a complete spinal evaluation. She suggested that I make an appointment with the doctor.

By this time, I would have seen anyone because I was so "sick and tired, of being sick and tired" and putting up with the pain and struggling to breathe.

At my first appointment with Dr. Duane, I was surprised to learn that my spine was not correctly aligned. I knew that my posture was poor; but didn't realize the connection to my health. I began to attend Dr Duane's health-care classes and learned about the human body and how it functions. After beginning chiropractic care, I noticed my condition was improving. For the first time in years, my knees did not ache all night. I was able to run for longer periods and my breathing came easier.

Within the first year under chiropractic care, my knees felt great and I no longer needed an inhaler. My tension headaches cleared up and my regular bouts of cold symptoms disappeared. I also noticed that I was able to relax easier, my concentration improved, and my academic marks increased.

To say the least, I questioned the link between my improved health and chiropractic. I knew that nothing else had changed. I had introduced chiropractic into my life, my subluxations were being corrected, and my overall health was improving. Yes, there was and continues to be a direct link between my great health and chiropractic.

I was blown away by my introduction to chiropractic and wanted to be a part of it for the rest of my life. My injuries provided me the opportunity to find my purpose in life: to help others discover optimal health. I continue to enjoy educating others on how they can reach their health potential and get the most out of their lives.

In my first year in practice, I met my wife, Brandi. Together we came up with the kitchen sink analogy and created a website—www.howisyoursink.com—to help our patients and the world devise strategies that can support their chiropractic care and improve their health for the rest of their lives.

Following is Brandi's personal discovery of health and well-being through chiropractic.

## Why I Became a Chiropractic Advocate

Brandi MacDonald

Chiropractic presented itself to me long before I was familiar with its Art, Science and Philosophy. I was born into a small

Metis community in Northern Alberta. The Metis people have long since known that the land that was once so good to them, no longer holds the same promise. Their Cooperatives, most look like a developing country, are community like dwellings. Destitute poverty and lack of vision, direction, and social status have not boded well for my people. One can only imagine the trauma on the general population's health.

I was born to a fourteen-year-old child/mother, who had the foresight to realize that this was not an environment in which I was destined to live. She gave me the greatest gift by putting me up for adoption. I spent the first three months in foster care, before I was placed with my adoptive family, whom I call my family today.

From the beginning, my health was precarious. I remember drinking black syrup called iron, because of anemia. I remember being told what a great baby I was because I slept for long periods of time. When I was eight or nine, because of chronic tonsillitis, I had to get my tonsils removed. I was underweight for my age, which was a primary concern for the doctor. I nearly bled to death after the tonsillectomy and my incisions had to be cauterized numerous times. During recovery, my mother held my hand because they were concerned about my racing heart as I came out of the general anesthetic.

From a young age, I remember believing that sickness was an event in my life that was uncontrollable. I was its victim. As I grew older, I continued to solidify this belief system. Every physician asked about my genetic pre-disposition to numerous diseases. And every time that question was posed, I shrank a little more into my sickness belief system, because I didn't have any information about my genetic pool.

Throughout high school, my "normal" illnesses continued. I got sick with every "normal" infection, cold, flu, impetigo, etc. I was diagnosed with chronic fatigue. The perfect sleeping baby was now a teenager who was exhausted all the time—for no apparent reason.

I failed every Canada Fitness Test because I couldn't do the 800-meter run around the track, and I couldn't engage my lower lumbar spine and core muscles to pull up and do even ONE sit up. When I was sixteen, I started to notice large lumps on my lower back, the lumbar spine. Eventually, I was unable to get out of bed in the morning without intense pain and stiffness. My mother took me to a physician who x-rayed my spine and told me I was born without one of the lower vertebrae. There was nothing I could do about it—except take more medication.

At the tender age of nineteen, I was diagnosed with cervical cancer. I went through treatment and came out the other end supposedly "healthy." At twenty-one, my bladder and kidneys started to fail. After chronic bladder and kidney infections and output issues, I was put through invasive testing to determine the cause. Nothing was found.

I continued taking anti-inflammatory, auto-immune suppressant, and antibiotic drugs. The physicians told me there was nothing wrong, so there was nothing much they or I could do—except continue taking the drugs.

In my mid-twenties, I met a chiropractor. Until then, I had not heard much about chiropractic let alone talk with a chiropractor. No one in my life had ever seen a chiropractor. In fact, like so many others, I was resistant and ignorant to chiropractic.

What little I thought I knew about chiropractic, was wrong. As I began to learn about the body's inborn ability to heal itself, and how the systems worked in harmony, the more I began to see the difference in my health ideology and the possibility for my future health. My kitchen sink was overflowing with the three stressors in the nervous system. Chemically, I was dependent on antibiotics, painkillers, and digestive medication. Physically, I could barely move to even turn my stress response off. Emotionally, I was exhausted.

I started chiropractic care and began to listen to the leaders of this magnificent profession. I was introduced to innate intelligence and universal intelligence, the nervous system, omeostasis, and the power of thought and healing. I began to earn how to both lessen the flow of water from the tap into my ink, as well as how to open up the drain. My health challenges vere still present, but gradually something started to change, ever o slightly. It was almost unnoticeable.

By far, the most significant change was my attitude. I had ope for a better life and a better future. After this change, everyhing else happened in perfect harmony. I began to see more and nore possibility. At twenty-eight, I started running—and ten nonths later I completed an ultra-marathon in the mountains. I ave since run four half-marathons. I also stopped all medication nd have been completely drug free for six years. I plan on being rug free for the rest of my life.

Every day I awaken and ask myself what I can do today to ustain and feed my soul. I ask more of myself and of my health ecause I know it is available. I no longer think of victimization.

I champion others to believe in themselves and in their health otential. People in some of the wealthiest and most advanced ountries are dying at alarming rates. Something needs to happen. n my humble opinion, after being a victim for so many years, the irst change that must take place is in our attitudes about health nd healing, and our ability to do something about it.

Chiropractic and chiropractors are best positioned to take center stage in this health-care revolution. The basic chiropractic philosophy is one of belief in the human body's innate ability to heal itself provided there is no interference. This theory has existed for centuries and was brought back to society in 1895 by the founder of chiropractic.

It is not too late to embrace this philosophy and re-dis cover your health and vitality. My chiropractic story is nc unique. True wellness lies at the heart of chiropractic—noth ing more, and nothing less.

If you would like more information on how to improv your health, please visit www.howisyoursink.com and sig up for our free "How is Your Sink" newsletter.

You can also e-mail or phone us at Whitemud Crossin Chiropractors:

www.whitemudcrossingchiropractors.com
Phone: 780-430-7549

Email:
drdon@shaw.ca
info@brandimacdonald.com

# 3.

# Ways of a Wellness Warrior

## Dr. Randy Koski, BSc, DC

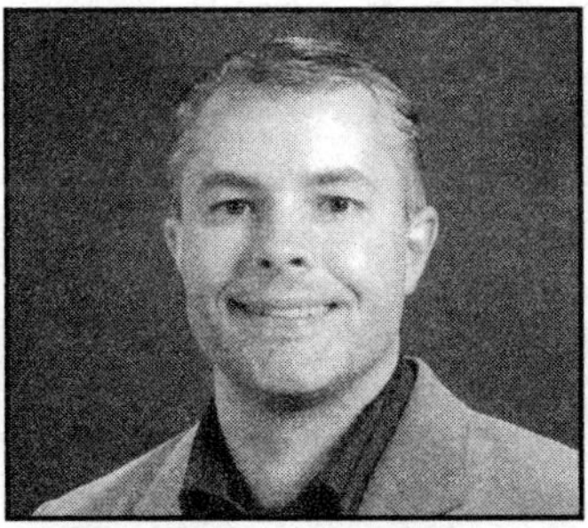

**Dr. Randy Koski** has a Bachelor of Science degree in chemistry. In 1996, he graduated summa cum laude from New York Chiropractic College with a Doctor of Chiropractic degree. During his time at NY Chiropractic College he served as president of the Canadian Chiropractic Club.

After graduation, he returned to his hometown of Sudbury, Ontario, to begin his career. He has since served as vice president of the Sudbury and District Chiropractic Society.

Dr. Koski has built two successful practices, where he serves his patients with kindness, love, and understanding. His clinic is a recognized externship clinic for chiropractic interns and, during the eleven years that he has been in practice, he has mentored many new graduates.

He is a knowledgeable and trustworthy chiropractic advocate and often speaks at schools, community groups, and businesses.

His passion and commitment to the health and well-being of the community that he serves has fuelled his search for the most current information on wellness. He has successfully completed the Six Advisors Coaching program and is currently pursuing a wellness certification.

Dr. Koski is a gentle, loving family man with a beautiful wife, Jodie, and an energetic toddler, Katie. He lives surrounded by his family and friends in the city of Greater Sudbury. He is involved in his community and has been a coach and trainer in minor league hockey. Dr. Koski continually strives for balance in life and is dedicated to helping others achieve the same.

> "Nobody has ever been able to scientifically prove that it is necessary to get sick."
>
> Deepak Chopra

## Introduction

Ever since I began my work as a chiropractor, I have seen the miracles of what the human body is capable of accomplishing when it is given purity and sufficiency. I have also witnessed the devastation of sickness and ill health when people are toxic and deficient in essential nutrients. My mission is to positively influence people's health and well-being through the delivery of exceptional patient-centered chiropractic wellness care. My team is fully dedicated to educate and serve the families of our community by providing them with the most up-to-date information on health and wellness. This involves providing physiologically compatible care by sharing what is essential to life, eliminating what is toxic, and ultimately creating purity and sufficiency that will allow their bodies to function at their God-given potential.

Eighteen years ago, when I began my journey to understand how the human body works and stays well, I could not have imagined the truly miraculous ways that a human body copes and adapts to everyday stressors. The following questions fueled my search: If we truly were meant to be healthy, why are so many people sick and dying prematurely? How do we get sick? What is this concept called "wellness?" Why don't doctors talk about and teach about keeping your health? What can we do if we have lost our health?

The answers to these questions form the basis of how my clinics are run and how my staff leads our patients on their journeys back to discovering and maintaining their health.

Unlike your car, truck, or household appliances, you did not come with an owner's manual at birth and you have no knowledge on how to troubleshoot when there is a challenge nor do you have a maintenance plan on how to keep your body functioning at its best. The general population receives little to no formal education or training on the most important subject that could ever be taught: their health!

For the most part, people rely on parents, family, friends, and worst of all, financially motivated advertising, for their health information. Very little accurate information on how the human body actually functions to stay well is readily available to the average person. In my opinion, this does not allow people to make informed choices regarding their health and wellness needs.

If you are *Tired of Being Sick and Tired,* this book is definitely for you.

During the last decade, I developed a keen interest in personal growth and development, which encompasses the wellness paradigm. My team stays current by attending conferences and seminars. Presently, as part of my continuing education, I am studying a wellness certification program to become a leader in the science of wellness.

In order to understand wellness, we need to define it. The Merriam-Webster online dictionary defines *wellness* simply: "The quality or state of being in good health especially as an actively sought goal."

Arizona State University (ASU) has a more comprehensive definition:

> "Wellness is an active, lifelong process of becoming aware of choices and making decisions toward a more balanced and fulfilling life. Wellness involves choices about our lives and our priorities that determine our lifestyles. The wellness concept at ASU is centered on connections and the idea that the mind, body, spirit and community are all interrelated and interdependent."

The National Wellness Institute definition is: "Wellness is an active process of becoming aware of and making choices toward a more successful existence."

Finally, this definition proposed by John W. Travis, MD:

"Wellness is a choice—a decision you make towards optimal health. Wellness is a way of life—a lifestyle you design to achieve your highest potential for well-being. Wellness is a process—a developing awareness that there is no end point, but that health and happiness are possible in each moment, here and now. Wellness is a positive acceptance of oneself. Wellness is the interaction of the body, mind and spirit—the appreciation that everything we do, think, feel, and believe has an impact on our state of health."[1]

This definition by Travis is probably the most encompassing definition I have found. From a practitioner perspective, this definition allows patients to become empowered and in control of their own health and lives.

Please take notice that there is no mention of *symptoms* in any of the above definitions. This is a gigantic leap from the medical model of sickness and disease care that proposes we are at the mercy of our genetic makeup and can, therefore, only watch and wait until we develop symptoms of a disease.

The allopathic model suggests that, as a disease consumes us, we can only attempt to medicate it or surgically remove it to slow it down. This is a disempowering and victimizing perspective, which truly is diametrically opposed to the health-and-wellness paradigm as described in chiropractic, as it focuses on taking care of oneself only when symptoms occur. When you stop to think about this, it makes little sense; but, nevertheless, this is the main focus of our present medical-care system, a system that tries to defeat anyone who presents a different model of healthcare.

Chiropractic is one of the most misunderstood professions. It evokes emotion when it is brought up in conversation, likely due to an enormous lack of understanding about what chiropractic truly represents. When people begin to understand what chiropractic stands for, I believe they will embrace chiropractic as a means to foster their journeys to wellness.

*Chiropractic*, taken from its Greek roots, literally means "done by hand." There are three components to chiropractic: the philosophy, the science, and the art. Although the core philosophy about how chiropractic views health and healing has never changed, the science behind what chiropractors stand for and what we do has evolved to a point that supports the core philosophical components of the discoverer of chiropractic, D. D. Palmer. The art of chiropractic refers to the techniques that are utilized to remove the deficiency of movement in the body and restore the communication between the brain and the tissue cells.

Most people have the common misperception that chiropractors are *bone* doctors, but actually we are *nerve* doctors. This will be explained clearly throughout the chapter.

In order to understand health, you must know how you developed. Every human being starts from two cells. When a sperm fertilizes an egg, a process that is nothing short of miraculous occurs. These two cells divide to form approximately eleven trillion cells. Yes, that is 11,000,000,000,000 cells. While going through this division process, specialization occurs and different organs and systems are created—the heart, lungs, kidneys, liver, stomach, nervous system, skin, muscles, bones, etc. Within thirty-seven weeks, these two cells become a human being.

Chiropractors understand that there is an inborn self-healing and self-regulating intelligence within every human being that expresses itself in fully functioning body systems. Your heart beats without you having to think about it. Your lungs breathe in vital air, your body digests food, and your brain processes millions of signals every second without you being consciously aware of it. These biological processes are designed for flawless execution every second of your life! Likewise, the chemicals your body produces are made in perfect amounts and when they are required.

Can you imagine having to think about which hormones, proteins, or enzymes to produce, or which chemical reaction to perform in order to survive? There is virtually a zero chance of that happening and, therefore, a zero chance that you would continue living if you had to think about all of these vital functions in order for them to occur!

The first structure that develops in a growing fetus is the master computer and its components. This system, referred to as the central nervous system, is composed of the brain and spinal cord (the extension cord from the brain). Beyond the spinal cord and part of the peripheral nervous system are thirty-two pairs of spinal nerves that travel from the spinal cord, exiting the spine to transfer information to and from all parts of the body. This makes up the majority of the nervous system, which is important to understand because the nervous system is responsible for controlling every function in your body.

Many people believe that the heart and blood system are the body's master controls. However, the truth is that everything that is put into and taken out of your blood is controlled by the nervous system. In fact, your heartbeat is controlled by the nervous system. The diameters of your blood vessels are controlled by the nervous system. No nervous system, no heartbeat; no heartbeat, no nutrition transport system—and, therefore, no life.

Every function of every system and part of your body is governed by the master system: the nervous system.

Our creator chose to enclose the entire central nervous system, brain, and spinal cord in bone. This is because they are fragile and vital to your existence. Your skull protects your brain and your vertebral column protects your spinal cord. Your vertebral column is also intelligently formed. It consists of twenty-four movable segments, called vertebra, that stack on one another. Each vertebra has a donut-shaped hole that leaves room for the spinal cord to pass through. Between each vertebra is a disc that provides cushioning for compressive type forces, the most common one being gravity.

Basically, the spine was designed to last a lifetime without wearing out!

Your spinal column is formed with three sixty-degree arcs; one of the most stable arc systems in nature. At the back of each vertebra are two joints that allow the spine to bend and twist. As each vertebra stacks on the next, there is a hole that is formed on the left and right sides. These openings provide room for nerves to exit the spinal column. The purpose of these spinal nerves is to provide the hard wiring for communication between the brain and the cells. The current that flows through the spinal nerves provides vital information to the organs, glands, immune system, skin, muscle, and bones. These nerves also provide the brain with vital information regarding how every part of the body is functioning. This process of communication is perfect as long as there is no interference.

The main focus of a chiropractor is to determine the presence of any interference in this vital communication.

For example, what would happen if the nerve that goes to the stomach is cut? The answer is simple: the stomach would not function. What if the nerve flow to the stomach is being interfered with, would the stomach run more or less efficiently? The answer is: less efficiently, of course.

If your stomach was running less efficiently for a long period of time, it could develop a problem such as an ulcer, couldn't it? And, before an ulcer actually forms, you might experience indigestion or other digestive difficulties.

If there is interference to the nerves that communicate with the lungs and bronchial system, a variety of respiratory disorders can occur, including but not limited to a commonly seen and quickly expanding condition called *asthma*. This process takes a long time to occur and you would not necessarily experience any symptoms while it is developing.

How can dysfunction occur without any pain, discomfort, or other noticeable symptom you ask? The answer is simply that less than ten percent of each nerve is capable of perceiving pain, so interference can exist and no pain will be felt; therefore you will believe you are healthy when, in fact, your body is in crisis. The chart below shows a cross-section of a spinal nerve. The part that supplies your organs and glands is not able to perceive pain. Also, the part that supplies your muscles is not able to perceive pain. You can have interference to the nerve for a long period of time (months or years) before you feel the effects of the organ or gland not functioning properly and manifesting in sickness.

Another result of interference to the spinal nerve(s) is how the body communicates with the brain. According to Dr. James Chestnut, when there is a tissue injury, your body SCREAMS to the brain, through the nervous system, that help is needed. The brain then initiates what is called a *stress response, adrenaline rush,* or a *fight-or-flight response.* Whatever you choose to call it, the body intelligently goes into defense mode. It releases two hormones—adrenaline and Cortisol—that get the body ready for survival. The following actions will occur;

- Increased heart rate
- Blood vessels constrict
- Increased blood pressure
- Increased blood sugar levels
- Increased blood fat (lipid) levels
- Increased blood cholesterol (high LDL and low HDL)
- Increased blood clotting factors (just in case you are wounded)

# FEELING VS. FUNCTION

There are three parts of the central nervous system:

1) **MOTOR NERVES** (control muscles)
2) **AUTONOMIC NERVES** (control blood vessels, organs, and glands)
3) **SENSORY NERVES** (transmit pain)

Notice on the graph below that the sensory part, which transmits pain, is only a small portion of the central nervous system. Nerve root compression can exist without pain.*

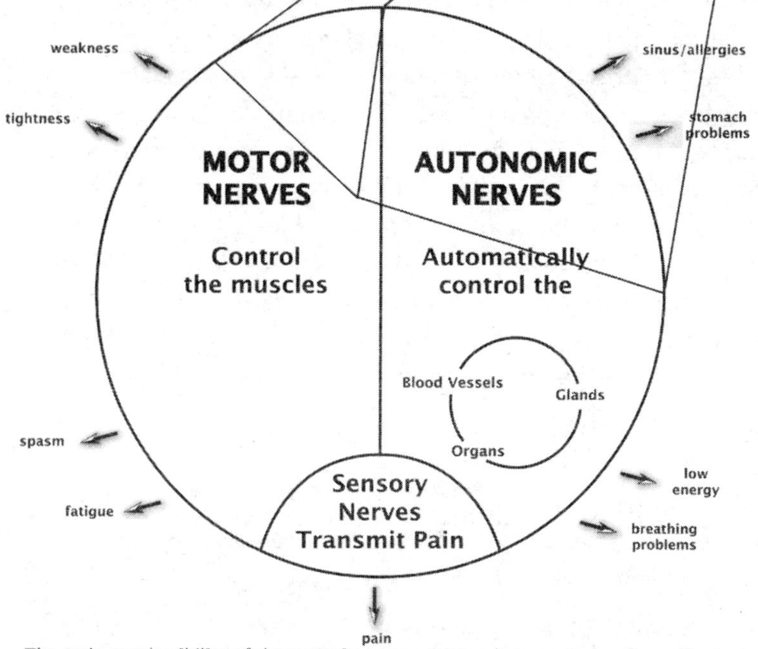


The main responsibility of the central nervous system is to control and coordinate the function of your entire body, plus adapt and relate to its environment.

* Hause M: Pain and the nerve root. Spine 1993; 18(14):2053.

- Increased protein degradation of muscle and connective tissue
- Insulin resistance
- Increased feelings of stress, fear, anxiety, and depression
- Decreased short-term memory, concentration, and ability to learn new material
- Decreased Serotonin levels—it is being used in other pathways
- Increased sensitivity of sensory systems, including those for pain
- Decreased cellular immunity
- Decreased anabolic (growth) hormones—growth hormone, testosterone, luteinizing hormone
- Bone loss, muscle-fiber type changes[2]

The human body is capable of adapting to stressors for the short term. The stress response is designed to get you away from an immediate threat, such as meeting a bear in the woods. After the short-term threat is over, however, your body is supposed to stop responding to the stress. The stress response is not meant to go on day after day or year after year, which is why our nervous systems have not adapted well to the chronic stress that is pervasive in most people's lives.

The long-term effects of stress (physical, chemical, or emotional) are summarized in the chart on page 50.

That's right. Long-term stress and a nervous system that is in acute disarray can lead to heart disease, depression,

# DISEASES OF ADAPTATION

| | |
|---|---|
| 1. Increased heart rate, blood pressure, fatty acids, glucose, clotting factors → | **Heart Disease** |
| 2. Decreased serotonin, increased noradrenaline → | **Depression; Fatigue; Anxiety; Memory, Learning, and Attention Deficits; Accelerated Aging (lack of growth hormone)** |
| 3. Insulin receptor resistance and increased glucose and lipids → | **Obesity and Type II Diabetes** |
| 4. Increased Cortisol → | **Chronically suppressed immune function and loss of bone density** |

fatigue, anxiety, memory loss, learning and attention deficits, accelerated aging, obesity, Type II diabetes, and a chronically suppressed immune system which predisposes you to many other illnesses. These conditions are diseases of adaptation. They are not the genetic miscues as some people would have you believe.

Here is a personal story that helped me understand this.

Fourteen years ago, my mother developed heart disease and had bypass surgery. At that time, we knew (or thought we did) that heart disease ran in the family and we believed there was no way to avoid it.

The cardiac grafts are only supposed to last ten to twelve years. So, with every annual checkup, the stress and emotion were intense. We wondered: will more blockage be found? Will further surgery be required? We knew that every surgery presents possible complications, and sometimes devastating effects, so we walked on egg shells whenever Mom had her annual consultation.

Well, the news that came out of the specialist's mouth this year was not what anyone expected to hear: "There are no blockages in the arteries around your heart. Everything is clear. I do not need to see you anymore."

Obviously those words brought tears of joy to the family, me included. We were in shock; but full of wonderment. I had heard that heart disease is reversible—and now I knew someone whose body had intelligently rid itself of the disease!

It has been three years since we received this news, and my mother's health continues to remain great.

How did this happen? I will let you know after I give you vital information so that you can better understand the process for "lack of health."

## Causes of Nervous System Interference

The most common cause of interference to the spinal nerve is *vertebral subluxation*. The simple definition is: "a misalignment of a vertebra that results in interference to the impulse that travels from the brain through the spinal nerve to the cell, and from the cell to the brain."

The consequences of vertebral subluxation cannot be overstated. It will most assuredly result in abnormal function in the part of the body that the nerve supplies AND it will activate the stress response.

A more detailed definition involves five components and is referred to as the *Vertebral Subluxation Complex* (VSC).

1. Loss of normal position (or alignment) of each vertebra leads to restricted movement.
2. Abnormal positioning can lead to shortened muscle tissue with decreased strength and flexibility, as well as to scar tissue development.
3. Interference to the spinal nerve.
4. Swelling or inflammation may develop in the disc, joints, or surrounding tissues.
5. Degenerative Joint Disease (known as DJD or osteoarthritis) may occur in the affected area leading to the development of bone spurs.

VSC is silent—unless you are lucky enough to have it irritate a part of the nerve that can perceive pain (remember that is less than 10% of the nerve). The fact that VSC does not usually involve pain until much later in the process is why most people live with vertebral subluxation for a long period of time and their spines will show signs of degeneration, sometimes at a very young age, before it is discovered.

Spinal degeneration/decay occurs when there is a mechanical imbalance over a long period of time. A common scenario is that patients feel pain while simply bending over. When they visit a chiropractor, they explain that their back just "gave out" on them. This happens because they didn't realize they had a problem long before they felt any pain. They also didn't know that the spine requires maintenance.

The most important job I have as a chiropractor is to teach people how to maintain their spine once correction has occurred. There are four components to spinal maintenance: proper posture, enough water (up to eight large glasses per day, preferably purified), exercise, and regular spinal check-ups to determine if your spine has VSC.

Checkups are vital to maintenance because VSC doesn't commonly cause pain and typically it activates the stress response silently.

There is wonderful research that describes the detrimental effects of spinal subluxation and nervous system disturbance on organ system function and human health and well-being, as well as research that describes the beneficial effects of spinal subluxation correction. Ronald Pero, PhD, chief of cancer prevention research at New York's Preventive Medicine Institute and a professor of medicine at New York University, performed one of the most important studies showing the positive effect chiropractic care can have on the immune system and general health. Dr. Pero measured the immune systems of people under chiropractic care as compared to those in the general population and those with cancer and other serious diseases. In his initial three-year study of 107 individuals who had been under chiropractic care for five years or more, the chiropractic patients were found to have a 200% greater immune competence than people who had not received chiropractic care, and 400%

greater immune competence than people with cancer and other serious diseases. The immune system superiority of those under chiropractic care did not diminish with age.

Dr. Pero stated: "When applied in a clinical framework, I have never seen a group other than this chiropractic group to experience a 200% increase over the normal patients. This is why it is so dramatically important. We have never seen such a positive improvement in a group ..."[3]

## Causes of VSC

Who should be checked by a chiropractor or, better yet, who should recruit a chiropractor to be a part of their health-care team? Before I answer this question, let's identify the causes of VSC.

The number one cause of VSC appears to be improper posture. If postural imbalances are not identified and corrected they create stress on the spine and interference to the nervous system. It is my experience that this problem is of epidemic proportion and often begins at a very young age. And, the reason appears to be simple: lifestyle.

Examples of pathological lifestyle habits include the use of walkers and jolly-jumpers at a time when the child's spine and nervous system are not yet ready to be erect for extended periods of time, the intensive use of video games with forward head posture, watching television, sitting for long periods of time, and simply lack of movement and exercise. Also, what is considered a natural birth process is a common cause of VSC. Most babies examined by chiropractors have problems in their necks and pelvic areas from birth trauma.

Delivering a baby in the semi-reclined position causes this. My daughter was checked minutes after she was delivered and I contend that every baby should have a spinal checkup as soon after birth as possible. If a newborn has VSC at the level of the first bone in the spinal column (called the atlas or first cervical vertebra) and the subluxation is left uncorrected, over time developmental problems may become evident.

As reported in the *Manuelle Medizin*: "Traumatization of the suboccipital structures (upper neck vertebrae) inhibits functioning of motor development. These children may only show minor symptoms in the first months of their life. Later on, at the age of 5 or 6 they begin to suffer from headaches, postural problems or diffuse symptoms such as sleep disorders, being unable to concentrate, etc. Adjustment of the occipito-cervical region leads to the disappearance of problems that the parents have not reported because they have never seen any connection with the vertebral spine."[4]

According to prominent manual specialist G. Gutmann, from Bad Sassendorf, West Germany, blocked nerve impulses at the atlas may cause many clinical features from central motor impairment to lower resistance to infection—especially ear, nose, and throat infections. From this and other German medical studies, Gutmann concluded that approximately 80% of all children are not in autonomic balance and that many have atlas blockage or subluxation."[5]

There are many other studies that support his findings, but most important are the testimonials given by patients who notice their children do not get the usual colds or ear infections when they are getting checked and adjusted regularly. Such situations are easily corrected and prevented. The corrective force required is extremely gentle and is nothing more than a vibration of a skilled finger in the appropriate area. Most babies actually sleep through their adjustments.

Here is another interesting and true story. We met Janet's (name changed to maintain patient confidentiality) mom and baby brother first. Janet's mom often talked to me about her young daughter who has autism. Finally, Mom decided to give chiropractic a try for Janet. She knew that chiropractic care helped her throughout her pregnancy and her son after he was born. She hoped that chiropractic could make a difference for her daughter.

Janet's autistic behavior made visits to our clinic interesting. She didn't like to be touched, and she was loud and moved fast—all of which proved to be challenging. We started slowly. First, Janet was allowed to walk around freely. Eventually she entered the adjusting rooms, and then she actually touched the exam tables. Finally, one day, she got up on the adjusting table and I was able to assess her spine. I quickly moved to adjusting her subluxations and, eventually, Janet was so comfortable with everyone at the clinic she actually made eye contact with some of the team. Getting adjusted became very natural for her.

One day, her mom came in and told us that Janet had been to her family doctor and she had climbed up on the exam table, lay face down, and let him check her ears and throat. At first, we did not understand the significance of this event until Janet's mom explained that this was the first time Janet was examined by the family doctor *without being sedated*! Mom could not thank us enough for the difference chiropractic had made in Janet's life.

The most significant milestone with Janet took place one day when she was waiting for her checkup. Janet began to sing—something she had never done before. That day every member of our team wiped tears from their eyes! And, to this day, Janet continues to have regular chiropractic adjustments, as does the rest of her family.

Another common cause of VSC is physical trauma that you experience throughout your life. Poor posture, a slip and fall, a motor vehicle accident, and anything in between can cause VSC. I have read that the average toddler has four thousand falls by the age of five! Do you think that any number of these can affect the spine and cause VSC? The answer is absolutely yes!

I have a recent story to share with you. Mr. James (name changed to maintain patient confidentiality) came to our clinic at the suggestion of his wife, who has been a patient for some time. He is a funny, smart, gallant gentleman in his eighties. I did the initial consultation and exam and, after a report of findings, he started his plan of care. Mr. James was responding well to the adjustments and, after several months of care, was fast approaching conversion to a maintenance schedule of care.

One day, he stepped aside at the top of some stairs to let a lady pass by, lost his balance, and tumbled to the bottom. He was unable to come to the clinic and missed a couple of appointments. His wife told us about the accident and expressed concern for him. He was becoming disoriented and, although he had been examined by his family doctor after the fall, they could find nothing broken and no particular reason for any type of intervention. One morning, Mrs. James realized that her husband was not himself. She called the clinic to see if we could help. My chiropractic assistant responded: "Of course, come in right away." Mrs. James was concerned about getting her husband to the clinic alone, so we met them at the car and assisted Mr. James into the clinic. At that time, he did not know where he was, he was unsure of his name, and didn't remember our names. He was unsteady on his feet, but appeared to feel safe in our environment.

After a thorough examination, I detected subluxations and adjusted him. After the adjustment, he sat up on the table and joked with me as usual. He left the adjusting room on his own steam, was walking with little assistance, and he joked with "the girls" at the front desk.

We still see Mr. and Mrs. James regularly for adjustments and we will always remember the day when Mr. James was returned to us! This is an example that you are never too old to take care of your spine and nervous system.

Emotional stress that you experience in everyday life can also cause VSC. According to Robert Hartman PhD, and as related in the *Six Advisors Coaching Academy Manual*, the average person has about 12,000 thoughts per day. Deep thinkers have about 50,000 thoughts. Your thought processes are the fuel behind your feelings, emotions, actions and behavior.[6] It is a fact that negative, stressful, and disempowering thoughts create a physical response in your body that can have negative effects over time. This can cause VSC, and also activate the stress response.

## Identifying and Correcting VSC

During an initial visit to our office, our goal is to identify whether you have vertebral subluxations. This involves taking a complete history to identify past traumas, lifestyle behaviors, and any other stressors. We also identify any toxicities or deficiencies that might be disallowing proper function.

An examination is then performed using orthopedic and neurological testing, postural analysis, and an assessment of spinal joint mobility through palpation or feeling joint motion. X-rays may be taken to determine the degree of structural abnormality or amount of spinal decay. Finally, a nerve scan is completed. This involves a series of five tests. We utilize this technology because it provides the best objective measurement of nerve interference. Remember, you can only tell the doctor if the part of the nerve that perceives pain is irritated, but cannot relate dysfunction in other parts of the nerves that send vital information to the organs, glands, immune system, or blood vessels. Following performance of a baseline scan, we continue to monitor function and progress with this same technology.

After the tests are completed and the information is collected, you receive a report of findings. This report has verbal and written components. It is designed to explain what the problem is, where it is, and what is required to improve your health status. The correction of VSC utilizes gentle and safe spinal adjustments, stretching, and therapeutic exercise to help hold adjustments and facilitate healing. The time that is required for the process of correction and return to health is dependent on how long you have had VSC. It stands to reason that the longer VSC has been present, the longer it takes to correct.

After subluxations have been corrected, there are four main actions required for proper care of your spine. Even though these have already been stated, they deserve repeating: drink plenty of water (at least eight tall glasses daily, preferably filtered water), specific postural exercises, proper ergonomics (correct posture while working, sitting, standing, laying down), and most importantly, spinal checkups to determine the presence of subluxations followed by immediate adjustment, even if there are no symptoms present.

There are three main components to keeping your health so that you can live life to the potential that you were designed to experience. Dr. James Chestnut, a leader in the field of health and wellness, simplifies these items: eat well, move well, and think well. These are the core lifestyle habits that my mother utilizes—and these habits have allowed her body to heal heart disease. Regular spinal adjustments are a key ingredient to the move well component of my mother's lifestyle changes and her journey to wellness.

By eliminating toxicity and deficiency in your life you, too, can BE WELL! You can live a life devoid of illness and truly live up to your full health potential. The most important action that you can implement to achieve this level of health and wellness is to stay informed and learn about health. Choose a wellness professional that can be your health coach for life, and experience the benefits of this partnership.

At Koski Chiropractic Clinic, we are here to serve you and would be honored to be your family chiropractor and health coach. Please contact us at Koski Chiropractic Clinics:

1177 Barrydowne Road, Suite 101
Sudbury, Ontario P3A 3V4
705-566-0723
drkoski@bellnet.ca

3249 Errington St.,
Chelmsford, Ontario P0M 1L0
705-855-8588

## Chapter Notes

1.Travis, John W., MD, www.thewellspring.com

2. Chestnut, James L., B.Ed., M.Sc., DC, *The 14 Foundational Premises for the Scientific and Philosophical Validation of the Chiropractic and Wellness Paradigm*, The Wellness Practice, 2003.

3. Pero R., "Medical Researcher Excited By CBSRF Project Results," *The Chiropractic Journal*, August 1989; 32.

4.Gutmann, G. "Kinematic Imbalances Due to Suboccipital Strain in Newborns," *Manuelle Medizin*, 1992.

5. Gutmann, G. *Manuelle Medizin*, 1982

6. Hartman, Robert PhD, *The Six Advisors Coaching Academy Manual*, 2007.

# 4.

# 5 Steps to Exceptional Health

## Dr. Ernest Li

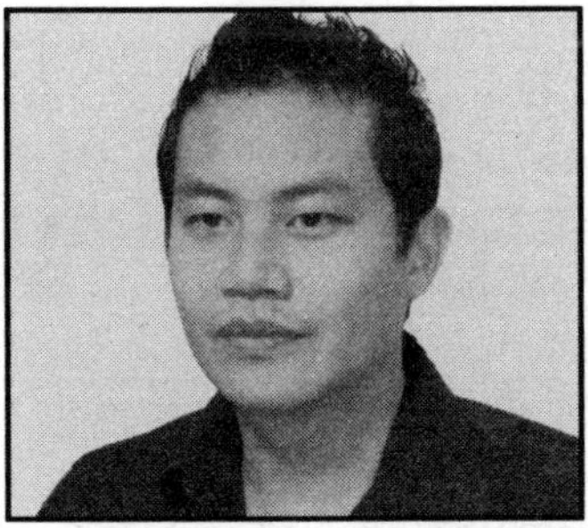

**Dr. Ernest Li** is a chiropractor who focuses on patient empowerment in the areas of health and personal development. He believes that there are many factors that cause pain involving the physical, mental, and spiritual planes. Ever since he discovered his purpose as a healer and leader in the field of chiropractic, he has been expanding his own knowledge in pursuit of mastering the seven areas of life: physical health, family, mental, career, social, financial, and spiritual.

His research and studies have taken him all over the world. He prides himself on his continual quest of self-mastery as a chiropractor, leader, author, husband, and father. He believes that his life purpose is to help people discover their full potential. He accomplishes this in his role of chiropractor and he will continue to strive to improve his skills, education, and communication skills to ultimately serve his patients and clients to the fullest extent possible. As a leader in his profession, Dr. Li continues to bring the message of health and chiropractic to as many people as possible.

Dr. Li was born and raised in Nova Scotia. He moved to British Columbia to attend Simon Fraser University. He completed a four-year Bachelor of Science degree in Kinesiology, as well as a two-year Health and Fitness Program. While attending university, he was involved in six motor vehicle accidents over a three-year period, which resulted in chronic pain in his neck and back. His treatment protocol included painkillers, physiotherapy, massage therapy, cortisone injections, and therapy at the Canadian Back Institute. Unsatisfied with his progress, coupled with the side effects of the medications, he decided to take his health into his own hands. His health took a turn for the better when, against his medical doctor's advice, he sought treatment from a chiropractor.

Dr. Li learned about the chiropractic philosophy that emphasizes the body's self-healing and self-regulating abilities. He was told that the repeated motor vehicle accidents caused his spine and neck to become misaligned, resulting in nerve compression that made his muscles constantly spasm and ache. The x-rays, the first set ever taken, confirmed four misalignments and a reversed curve in his neck. He was impressed by the chiropractic doctor's thorough consultation, examination, and diagnosis, and his commitment to treat the cause of the problem instead of just the pain.

The chiropractor suggested a treatment plan of several chiropractic adjustments over a number of months to correct the misalignments. Within three months, the pain and discomfort were gone. Dr. Li initially had dreams of becoming a medical doctor; but was so impressed by the effectiveness of the chiropractic care after other methods had failed to offer him relief, he chose to enroll in chiropractic school upon graduation from Simon Fraser. Dr. Li graduated from the Los Angeles College of Chiropractic in 2004 and started his own practice.

Today, he is the proud owner of two clinics, Heath Star Chiropractic and LUX Chiropractic. Every day Dr. Li is astonished to witness the magnificence of the human body. Every day he is more and more amazed at how the body can recover and thrive under the right circumstances. Most of all, he remains truly grateful for the opportunity to work with countless people and witness the power of the body's innate intelligence and its ability to self-regulate and heal. He is committed to his patients and his work as a chiropractor. Under no circumstance, will he ever take his work lightly because he believes that there is nothing more important to a person than his or her health.

> "A healthy body and healthy mind lead to a healthy spirit and a life lived to the optimum. Chiropractic helps people achieve all of this."
>
> Dr. Ernest Li

## Introduction

**A**re you familiar with the concept that anything that you believe is missing in your life, you tend to chase? In other words, the perceived voids create your values in life.

As a child, I was obese; and as a young man, I suffered chronic pain for over three years. So, for the majority of my life, up to that point, I was not very healthy. Eventually, I realized health was missing in my life, and it became a value and priority for me. I started to study health and fitness, both at school and at home. I voraciously studied the human body and the functions of the organs and muscles.

Learning about nutrition and exercise made an enormous impact in my life and allowed me to lose weight and become healthy. Today I realize that I had to lose my health first before it became important to me. In other words, my void became my passion. And, I see this pattern every day as a chiropractor.

Let me explain.

The average age of a typical chiropractic patient in my office is forty-two. The most common reason that my patients initially seek care is for chronic pain relief. More specifically, neck pain, headaches, and back pain. I have also realized that they have tried many different pills, therapies, and remedies prior to consulting me. So, it is safe to say that most patients requesting an appointment in my office are coming in as a last resort. As with all of my patients, I conduct a thorough history and physical examination and perform or refer out for the required diagnostic tests. When I review the findings, I am often astounded by the number of patients who have developed severe spinal degenerative disease—meaning that their true problems have been progressing for years without any signs.

With that said, I have found that there are two huge mistakes that people make regarding their health. The first mistake is that they usually wait until there is chronic pain before consulting a health-care provider. This is often a serious problem, because by the time there are signs and symptoms, there may already be permanent damage to the body. It would be like brushing your teeth or going to the dentist only when your teeth hurt. You know it is important to maintain your dental hygiene, but did anyone ever tell you that your spinal hygiene is even more important to maintain?

The second biggest mistake that people make about their health is that they fail to take proactive measures to maintain their bodies when they are healthy. I contend that pain is, in fact, a poor indicator of your overall level of health and that everyone should maintain their bodies while they are at their healthiest. It doesn't make any sense to wait until you lose your health before you start to care about it. When it comes to health, too many people function as described in the quote below.

> "If it ain't broken, don't try to fix it"
>
> Anonymous

There are five keys to long-lasting exceptional health. These steps will help increase your health and vitality for years to come. I have personally improved my overall health and fitness by following these steps, so it is possible to have better health as you age.

No matter where you are in terms of your health, by making a life-long commitment to improving your health, you will ultimately succeed. A ten percent improvement every year for five years will yield a fifty percent improvement over that period of time. To succeed in achieving exceptional health, it is imperative you realize that health is always a work in progress, i.e., it is something that you must continually work on every day. There are no long-lasting quick fixes for your health. But, if you follow these easy steps you can achieve exceptional health for you and your family.

### Step #1: Know what exceptional health is and set clear goals.

If you were to build a house, would you just hire a builder and tell him to build it? Of course you wouldn't. You would provide him with a blueprint to follow. The clearer the details, the faster and more organized your new home will be built. You need to have a goal and a plan of action to accomplish something with predictability.

Before we discuss setting goals for your health, we must first define what health is and what pain is because most people incorrectly equate being pain-free to having good health. According to *Webster's Dictionary, health* is "a condition of wholeness to which all the organs are functioning at 100 percent." Alternately, the World Health Organization defines health as "an optimal state of physical, mental, and social well-being and not merely the absence of disease and infirmity."

> "Crystal clarity of the objective is job one for attaining success in life. To the degree there is fogginess, is the degree to which one will fail"
>
> Brian Tracy

Based on these definitions, health is measured by the body functioning well. So, what is pain then? Pain, as described by the International Association for the Study of Pain, is an "unpleasant sensory and emotional experience associated with actual or potential tissue damage." In other words, pain is your body's way of letting you know something is wrong.

Is pain a bad or a good thing? Let me answer this question with an example. If you could choose to get rid of your body's way of perceiving pain for the rest of your life, would you do it? If you answered yes, you would ultimately be getting rid of your body's way of communicating to you. That would be like driving down the road in your car with the engine light on and placing a piece of tape over it and pretending there is no problem.

Likewise, if I broke my left leg, there would be pain. If I tried to bear weight on the broken leg, the pain would increase. What if I took enough medication to numb the pain so that I wouldn't feel anything? Would that fix the problem? Of course not. What if I started to walk on it again? Would it cause more or less damage to my leg? More, of course. Simply put, if you ignore the symptoms without fixing the problem, the problem will not only cause more pain but is likely to cause more damage. So, pain is not a bad sensation. Pain is a warning sign and actually helps protect your physical body from further damage.

The common misconception that being pain-free equates to good health is the cornerstone to much of society's health problems. Fifty percent of all Americans will die from heart disease and another 33 percent from cancer. In both cases, people rarely feel any symptoms until the disease is full-blown. As a matter of fact, in half of the cases of heart disease, a sudden heart attack followed by death is the first and obviously the only sign. Your arteries could be clogged for decades and you won't feel a thing.

Do you know of anyone who appeared to be in good health, and all of a sudden died from a massive heart attack? Were they healthy? Of course not. The same can be said about cancer. By the time a person has noticeable symptoms, they may have only weeks to live.

Thus, waiting until your body hurts is definitely not the best approach to maximizing your health potential.

Now that we have clearly defined the role that pain plays in your overall health, you can begin to set some goals. First, how long would you like to live? Would you like to live until you are one hundred years old? I often ask people at my workshops, "How many of you would love to live until you are one hundred years of age?" Not surprisingly, very few hands go up in the room. I then follow up with two questions: "Why would you not like to live to be one hundred?" and "How do you visualize a one-hundred-year-old person?" Common responses include: old-age homes, a loss of independence, wheelchairs, walkers, bed-ridden, diseases, and multiple medications and pills.

I then rephrase my question: "How many of you would love to live to be one hundred if you had good health?"

Not surprisingly, every hand goes up. The reality is, people are afraid of aging because of the growing statistics in North America that show that the average sixty-five-year-old takes eight to ten different medications; and that one out of three people over sixty-five will become permanently disabled.

By making your health a priority, that is by spending time, energy, and money on developing and maintaining your health, you can live a long life with vitality.

At the turn of the last century, the average life expectancy was forty-eight years of age. Now, the life expectancy is over eighty; and by 2020, it is said that the fastest growing age group will be people in their nineties.

Today, technology allows people to live much longer, but often with little quality of life. Life is not only about survival; it is the *quality* of life that is of great importance.

For instance, I have a patient who has been disabled since the age of fifty-five. If she lives until she is ninety, she will spend her last thirty-five years in a wheelchair. Even though she may be grateful to be alive, the quality of her life will continue to decrease.

What kind of quality is experienced by people who spend the last years of their lives fighting a terminal disease?

Everyone should have a goal to live to at least ninety, with their body functioning as well as it did in their twenties. Is this possible? Of course it is. What about genetics, you ask. It is reported that genetics have less than a 20 percent influence on your life expectancy while 80 percent of your quality of life is due to your lifestyle. This means that you can definitely control your destiny when it comes to your health. Therefore, everyone should set a clear goal to live to at least ninety, disease free and having a fully functioning body.

How do you want to look as you age? What shape do you want to be in? How much do you want to weigh? These are questions that should be addressed as you implement action steps as to how you will achieve success in health. Plan your diet as well as your physical activities. If you do not make a conscious effort to do something daily for your health, you will most likely not get around to it.

Visualize how you want to age. Picture yourself golfing or dancing in the Bahamas at ninety. Change the perception of old age. You can choose to have exceptional health for the rest of your life.

Write down affirmations about your exceptional health and feed your mind with pictures of vitality. If you do not work on your health, your certainty for attaining it is drastically reduced. Sit down and write objective and measurable goals for your health. Think about body weight, body fat percentage, blood pressure, and cholesterol. Implement daily exercise and stretching as action steps. Maintain your physical body by getting your teeth, eyes, and spine checked regularly. Set a time frame for the completion of your goals and review them regularly.

Hire a health coach to keep you accountable for your

actions. Select health-care professionals who are health-conscious themselves and who understand the concept of wellness, and then listen to their advice. Remember, your daily habits determine your destiny. Whatever you have done in the past to maintain your health has created the level of health that you enjoy today—and your actions today, will determine your health for tomorrow. If you are presently unhealthy, see yourself developing new habits on your road to recovery and, after you achieve the health that you want, always maintain it at its highest state by being proactive.

**Step #2: Maintain optimal spine and nerve function.**

Your spine allows your body to move. It helps keep you upright and it houses your lifeline—the spinal cord. Since you now have a clear goal of living to at least ninety, while maintaining full bodily function, it only makes sense to keep what runs your body in optimal shape. The brain and spinal cord make up your nervous system which controls and coordinates every function in your body. In fact, it is estimated that there are over three trillion bits of information being exchanged between the brain and the body each second!

> "First and foremost, look to the spine for the cause of disease."
>
> Hippocrates

The brain and spinal cord control your body both consciously (voluntarily) and unconsciously (involuntarily). Consciously, your brain can tell your arm to flex or your mouth to smile. It controls your ability to walk, move, and talk. Unconsciously, your brain simultaneously controls your breathing, heart rate, digestion, hormones, reproduction, cell function, etc. Actually, you do not have conscious or voluntary control over most of your body.

The brain and spinal cord are the only organs in the human body that are fully encased in bone. (The designer of your body definitely wanted to protect these vital organs.) The spine consists of twenty-four moveable vertebral bones and a fused sacrum and coccyx (tail bone). Seven cervical or neck bones, twelve thoracic or mid-back bones, and five lumbar or lower-back bones make up the spine. The spinal cord is contained within the spine. Nearly every nerve in the body is somehow connected to the spinal cord. The nerves exit through holes of the vertebrae called the IVF or Intervertebral foramen. A cushioning disc separates each vertebra. The spine is primarily responsible for movement of the body and the protection of the spinal cord, the lifeline of the body.

When the spine is in perfect alignment, the spinal cord and nerves are positioned in the most optimal biomechanical place. The brain, in this normal position, is able to send the trillions and trillions of messages to every organ, tissue, and cell of the body optimally. From the front, the spine should be straight. From the side, it is important that the spine have three curves, the cervical lordotic curve, the thoracic kyphotic curve, and the lumbar lordotic curve. When the spine misaligns, this creates compression on the spinal cord and nerves. We know that severe spinal injuries often result in the loss of muscle and organ function (paralysis).

For example, former actor Christopher Reeves fell off his horse and fractured his vertebra. The accident shifted his spine out of place by just over one centimeter, which was enough to permanently damage his spinal cord and nerves. Not only did he lose his ability to move, he also had diminished function to his organs and systems of his body. He could not breathe or defecate on his own. He eventually died from complications secondary to bed sores as a result of his spinal injuries.

We know that the spinal cord and nerves carry the power that keeps us alive and functioning well. What happens if you cut the nerve to a tooth? That's right, the tooth dies. What happens when nerves to organs are damaged? The organs slowly start to decrease in function and start breaking down, and eventually they start to die.

*Vertebral subluxation* is the term given to a misaligned vertebra that results in compression of the spinal cord and nerves. Acute causes of vertebral subluxations include falls, accidents, awkward twisting or bending, or trauma. Chronic causes include extended periods of sitting, poor posture, stress, and lifestyle.

How much abuse does your body take on a daily basis?

Since your bones and central nervous system do not feel pain, it may be difficult for you to know that you have vertebral misalignments present. Since we know that your structure often dictates your function, undetected spinal subluxations start to negatively affect nerve function to vital organs and invariably lead to dis-ease, and will cause progressive damage to the spine and its structures.

For example, a spinal misalignment left uncorrected for three to five years may not result in any pain or visible damage to the spine, even though there is nerve damage and dysfunction occurring. However, if left uncorrected for ten to twenty years, degenerative changes to the spine and its structures become evident. The longer a subluxation is left uncorrected, the more damage results.

It is like driving your car with its wheels out of alignment. The tires may have a life expectancy of 30,000 miles; but, their life expectancy decreases significantly when the wheels are not properly aligned. If the wheels are out of alignment, not only will the tires not last as long, but the function of the entire vehicle will be compromised. For instance, the car's fuel economy is less, the handling is worse, it vibrates more, you are likely to require premature replacement of wheel bearings, etc.

The same is true when your spine is not properly aligned. Research has shown that your spine is designed to last up to 140 years. However, your body and nervous system are compromised and the spinal structures will wear out faster if subluxations exist. Misalignments in your spine also compromise how your body functions by showing up as restrictions in your range of motion, uneven posture, cracking or popping sounds while you move and twist, tightness and tenderness. Since your brain controls your body by sending messages down the spinal cord and out through your nerves to your muscles and organs, subluxation may also interfere with your brain's ability to communicate with your body.

A spinal misalignment or subluxation will compress your spinal cord and nerve. This reduces the nerve supply to your muscles and organs, which is why spinal misalignments (vertebral subluxations) are so devastating; they interfere with how your body functions.

The nerves that exit your upper neck supply your head and control your ears, eyes, nose, and throat. Subluxations in the upper neck region may cause headaches, migraines, blurred vision, dizziness, ringing in the ears, tingling in the face, jaw pain, and difficulty swallowing.

The nerves that exit your lower neck control the muscles of your neck, upper trapezius muscle, shoulders, arms, and hands. These nerves also control the function of your thyroid gland, heart, and lungs. Subluxations in the lower neck region may cause neck, upper trapezius, shoulder, or arm stiffness, tingling, numbness, or pain.

The nerves that exit your thoracic or upper and mid-back region control the muscles in the back, in between the shoulders, chest, and abdominal area. Organs that are innervated or controlled from this area include the heart and lungs, the stomach, pancreas, liver, and gallbladder. Subluxations in this area commonly cause pain and stiffness in the upper and mid-back, tightness in between the shoulder blades, chest pain, heartburn, indigestion, and even acid reflux.

The nerves that exit your lower back region control the lower back, buttocks, thigh, and leg muscles. These nerves also control the bladder, bowels, reproductive organs, and kidneys. Subluxations in the lower back region may cause low-back pain, pain in the buttocks and legs, tingling, numbness, and radiating pain down the legs. Other symptoms may include increased frequency of urination, bowel and bladder trouble, bedwetting, painful menstruation, increased cramping, enlarged prostate, or even erectile dysfunction.

At my office, the initial goal is to diagnose the presence of vertebral subluxations, to assess the severity of any subluxations present, and to offer possible solutions to help you re-discover your health. Common objective tests for subluxation include a postural evaluation, range of motion testing, palpation, muscle testing following pertinent nerve distributions, high-tech computerized digital infrared thermography, and surface EMGs to measure nerve and muscle function. Plain film radiographic X-rays are then used to confirm the locations of vertebral subluxations and assess the severity of the damage to your spine. A normal x-ray will reveal no spinal decay or damage, proper curves from the side and a straight spine from the front. Diagnosed subluxations with a normal spinal x-ray are typically acute and are generally more easily corrected. A Phase One x-ray will reveal no spinal damage but will show altered curves from the side or from the front.

The most common abnormality is seen in the neck. The neck should have a C-shaped lordotic curve. This curve helps keep the alignment of the head and neck stable and allows for maximum nerve supply to the body. The most common alteration is a straightening or reversal of this curve. A straightened or reversed cervical curve will cause instability in the spine and a stretching effect on the spinal cord.

*Scoliosis* is a condition where the spine bends laterally or sideways. This condition usually starts in childhood and is due to an initial trauma, possibly during the birth process, a fall or an accident. This bending occurs because the child is in a growing phase. For example, if you bend a twig it will grow in the direction of the bend. If a Phase I subluxation is allowed to progress, it will lead to a Phase II. A Phase II x-ray will not only reveal abnormal spinal curves but also structural damage to the vertebra and disc. The disc is the cushion that is found between vertebra. Bone spurs, known as *osteophytes*, will form due to the abnormal stress of the misalignment and from the altered curves.

Discs degenerate or decay due to two main causes. The first has to do with blood supply. Discs have no direct blood supply and receive their nutrients through a process called *imbibition*. Imbibition pumps blood into the disc via movement. A spinal misalignment reduces and alters the normal spinal movement, therefore limiting this pumping effect and decreasing the amount of blood and oxygen that enters the disc, which leads to decreased disc health and ultimately decay of the disc and vertebra involved. A lifestyle that involves extended hours of sitting will also lead to more decay due to the lack of movement.

The second major reason discs degenerate is related to changes in the normal spinal curves. If someone is diagnosed with a Phase II x-ray, the subluxation is likely to have been present for ten to twenty years. Severe decay and spurring results in a Phase III x-ray, meaning the subluxation or misalignment has been present for twenty to forty years. Obviously we do not see Phase III X-rays in young children, and it is unfortunate to see many Phase III x-rays on relatively young adults who otherwise appear to be healthy.

When a patient is diagnosed with vertebral subluxation, the initial goal of care is to remove the compression off the spinal cord and nerves. Some chiropractors may call this initial phase the symptomatic relief phase, because by removing the pressure off the nerves, it often relieves the majority of pain or discomfort.

The primary method of accomplishing this is by a chiropractic adjustment. In this phase of care, the goal of the chiropractic adjustment is to restore normal nerve supply to the body. The adjustment is a very specific procedure that is remarkably safer than any other form of treatment, including medications. The frequency and length of treatment in this phase is primarily determined by the severity of the diagnosed subluxation. For example, it is much easier to remove the pressure off a spine that shows no degeneration versus one that has spinal degeneration or complications. The end of the initial phase is usually confirmed with a re-examination of the initial diagnostic tests. The positive tests should be negative at the end of this phase.

Once you have a normal x-ray of the spine, regular chiropractic checkups and adjustments are recommended to maintain proper alignment, to prevent premature wear or decay to the spine, and to maximize the nerve supply to your body. If you have any complicating factors, such as curve abnormalities or spinal damage, it is highly recommended to follow through with a program of spinal corrective care.

Corrective care techniques, such as Chiropractic Biophysics or Pettibon, are often used to correct subluxations, and, therefore, prevent any further damage to the spine and its structures. Correction of the subluxations allows the spine and body to function at their optimal levels. The techniques used in the corrective phase are similar to how dentists correct misaligned teeth by using braces, i.e., repetitive stress over a specific amount of time. The most common way of confirming the correction is by taking another X-ray.

After completing the corrective care, you will be invited to receive regular chiropractic checkups and adjustments. Choosing preventative and proactive care is the wellness way. If patients consider stopping chiropractic care once they start to feel well, I often challenge them with the following question: "Why would you spend all this time, effort, and money to correct your subluxations if you do not intend to *maintain* a normally functioning spine and nervous system?"

### Step 3: Exercise daily.

Researchers have discovered that human genes have not changed in over 30,000 years. What did humans do back then? They hunted and gathered all day long. They did not live a sedentary life, like most people do today. There were no televisions, video games, or computers that kept people glued to their seats. Humans did not have jobs that required them to spend up to twelve hours a day driving or sitting. The human body was designed to move and to be active.

Scientists have found that when wild animals are either domesticated or put into captivity, they die earlier and become fatter than their wild brothers and sisters, and are more depressed and have increased incidences of cancer.

Likewise, if we look at North America, society as a whole has never been sicker, more obese, or more depressed, and the cancer rates have never been as high.

Your body was designed to be active. Your spine was not designed to be sedentary for extended periods. Spinal discs get nourishment and blood supply through movement. Sitting in front of a computer with poor posture causes damaging changes to the curves of the neck and leads to premature degeneration.

Everyone should exercise at least twenty minutes every day. Research has shown that simply walking for twenty minutes per day can increase your quality of life and your life expectancy by up to six years!

### Step 4: Maintain a healthy diet.

In accordance with the fact that our genetics have not changed in over 30,000 years, we should also adopt a diet similar to that which we were created to eat. Since humans are hunters and gatherers by nature, we should eat food that we either hunt or gather.

I often tell my patients that they should eat anything they can hunt, pluck from a tree, or gather from the earth. Your body has the capability to easily digest foods that are free from preservatives and other manmade enhancements. It has the ability to break down and digest perishable meats and vegetables—but can it physically break down manmade chemicals and preservatives?

In North America, we demand our foods to be prepared fast and inexpensively. The only way the fast-food companies can give this to consumers is to make food last a long time and increase the speed of the cooking process—both of which eliminate most, if not all, of the nutrients while adding unhealthy chemicals

With the rates of obesity and diabetes reaching epidemic proportions, we must return to the foods that we were created to eat. Moderate portions of fresh meat, vegetables, fruits, and grains with as few preservatives as possible should be the staples of your diet. Supplement your diet with a high-quality multivitamin to ensure proper levels of minerals, vitamins, and anti-oxidants. Supplementing with fish oils is also important to keep adequate levels of omega 3 fatty acids in your diet. Omega fatty acids are only found in wild game and wild fish; and, since the majority of meats we consume today are farmed, it is essential to supplement with fish oils.

### Step 5: Reduce the stress in your life by creating balance.

Emotional stress is ultimately the primary cause of many bad habits and choices. Stress causes you to worry, stress may cause you to be emotionally unstable at times, and stress also causes your body's physiology to change.

For example, emotional stress can cause your body to be in a state of fight-or-flight (a sympathetic state). The fight-or-flight state increases your heart rate, reduces your rate of digestion, increases constipation, and changes hormone levels. Also, Cortisol levels increase with stress, which can lead to increased body fat storage and fatigue.

I have found the perfect formula to dispersing stress. It involves removing the fears or worries in your life and dissolving the guilt or resentment in your life. Without fear and guilt, you are left with a state that is truly you. Fear of insufficient finances, fear of loss, fear of rejection, and fear of acceptance can all lead to stress. Guilt from unethical behavior or resentment of past experiences also causes stress.

In a state of elation, you may not see any drawbacks. In a state of depression, you may not see any positives. There are always equal benefits and drawbacks to any situation. Realizing this helps create a true sense of balance. Reacting to events, when unbalanced, may cause you to become an exaggerated version of yourself. For instance, have you ever lost your temper and said things that you did not really mean? How did this benefit you and others around you? Not at all, right? When you choose to live in gratitude for who you are and what you have, you cannot live in fear, and you and others get to experience the best of who you are.

There are seven major areas you can choose to work on to reduce stress in your life. They include your mental self, family life, social life, career, finances, spiritual life, and physical health. To have a well-balanced life, all seven areas should be given attention.

It is estimated that eighty percent of all people spend their time, energy, and money on their top three areas. What this means is if you focus your time and energy on only three areas of your life, you will be weak in the other four areas.

For example, patients often tell me that their health is very important to them. I then ask them to describe a typical day, and they will tell me that they get up at six in the morning, leave for work, grab a coffee and a donut for breakfast, commute forty minutes, go to a fast-food restaurant for lunch, return to their job, commute forty minutes home, have dinner, and then watch television until bedtime. What they have told me is that they value their career, their finances, and their relaxation time (mental self). How much time did they actually dedicate to their health on this day? How much exercise did they get? Did they spend quality time with their family? Did they have time to count their blessings? Did they engage with others socially?

Juggling responsibilities is difficult. As part of my health coaching, I suggest that everyone dedicate time and energy to the important areas of their lives. Schedule time for exercise and stretching, meal planning, conversing with your family, etc.

Keeping a life schedule is important. If you plan something, it is more likely to happen. How much expendable time do you have on a daily basis? I have learned that if you do not make time for the priorities in your life, unimportant things will pop up to occupy your time.

You should consider your health to be your most crucial investment. Think about what would happen if you lost your health. Would it only impact you? No. How would it impact your family? Would it affect your finances? Would you be able to work? What if you became disabled? Hopefully, you get my point. Lose your health and every other important area in your life is dramatically affected.

When should you start investing in your health? My advice: right now. Maintenance of your body while it is at its healthiest is an investment that truly pays off. Make a commitment to discover what is possible for you starting today. Having a lot of money while having poor health doesn't make sense.

How do you know if you have a health problem? If you don't experience any symptoms, the smartest precaution you can take is to have a chiropractic checkup. Consider that most people have regular dental checkups. At some point, many of these people are told that they have a cavity. And, most of these people likely had no pain or other symptom to make them aware of the ensuing damages of the cavity.

During a routine dental checkup, the dentist discovered the cavity and prevented a more serious problem from developing. The same goes for your spine. Get your spine checked by a chiropractor as a pro-active step to ensure exceptional health. It could be the best investment you ever make.

I judge something's value by what happens if you lose it. If you lost your teeth, it could affect your quality of life; but if you lose the proper functioning of your spine and nervous system, it will definitely cause a loss of health and negatively affect your life—and your loved one's.

Chiropractic is an art, science, and philosophy that has impacted my life in tremendously positive ways—and it can impact your life, too. Remember, I came from a scientific background, and initially I was pessimistic and doubtful about any health-care field that wasn't considered mainstream. But, chronic pain, coupled with the side effects of multiple medications, introduced me to chiropractic. And through chiropractic, I have discovered faith in the human body and the human spirit and, ultimately, in our creator.

True healing comes from within, when the body is allowed to function at its fullest potential. Achieving this wellness state is possible by making the right choices about your health. Follow the five simple steps and live well and long and prosper. You were meant to thrive.

If I can assist you in any way as your health coach, please contact me at Heath Star Chiropractic in South Edmonton or at LUX Chiropractic in downtown Edmonton, Alberta via:

Email: ernestlidc@hotmail.com

Website: www.drernestli.com or

Telephone: 1-780-450-8854

# 5.

# TrueChiro Health Management

## Drs. Michel and Angel Dupuis

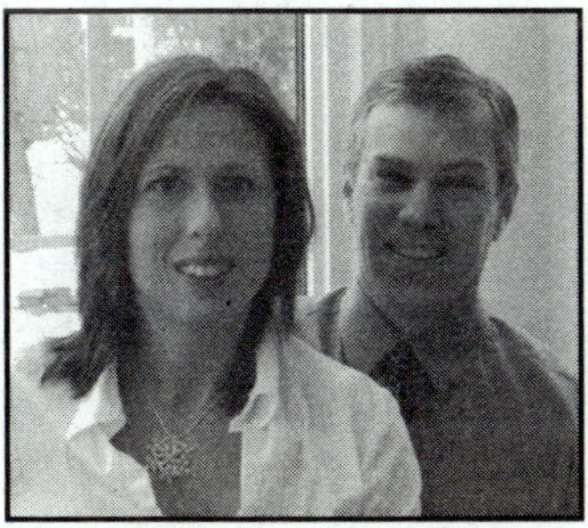

**Drs. Michel and Angel Dupuis,** a husband and wife team with a passion for helping people achieve their health goals, graduated from D'Arcy Lane Institute of Massage Therapy before attending Texas Chiropractic College, where they graduated summa cum laude. Dr. Michel was the class valedictorian and both received awards in the Omega Psi Honor Society and the 1998 All-American Scholars.

Currently Dr. Michel practices in New Liskeard at a fitness facility that incorporates rehabilitation and a Truestar Nutrition Center™. They believe that good food and nutrients help provide the right tools when integrated with a total program of healthcare. This total program includes work on the soft tissue (muscles, tendons, and ligaments), removing nerve interference through chiropractic, and rehabilitative exercise to promote positive long-term changes.

Drs. Michel and Angel are also in the process of developing a chiropractic diagnostic and treatment system to help chiropractors incorporate all the areas they believe are essential to providing a Total System for Health.

They reside in Northern Ontario, Canada, where they have owned three busy practices.

> "The doctor of the future will give no medicine but will interest his patients in the care of the human frame, in diet, and in the cause and the prevention of disease."
>
> Thomas Edison

Chiropractic patients are looking for information on their overall health. They want to know what they can do to stay healthy, what they should take, what exercises to do, and how to prevent injuries (subluxations) from reoccurring. Chiropractors have the knowledge, ability, and opportunity to provide their patients with this much-needed service.

We are on the cusp of a health-care revolution. Today's patients are the first generation to hold their health destinies in their hands.

There are four major forces behind this revolution:

**First** is an emerging awareness of the importance of exercise, nutrition, stress management, and chiropractic for long-term wellness.

**Second** is the aging population, with a baby boomer turning sixty every seven seconds.

**Third** is increased longevity.

And **fourth** is a shift in spending.

Healthy living and aging is a $480 billion industry with $125 billion being spent on relaxation and recreation; $105 billion on senior living and elder care; $66 billion on food, beverages, and supplements; $50 billion on fitness, weight loss, and wellness; $45 billion on complimentary and alternative medicines; $32 billion on technology, product development, and information; $30 billion on personal care; and $13 billion on substance abuse. By 2020, these expenditures will grow to over one trillion dollars. (North Castle Partners)

More than 33 percent of North Americans choose to treat their illnesses with alternative therapies. Chiropractic is the most common, followed by acupuncture, massage therapy, breathing exercises, herbal medicines, and meditation. In the United States, 158 million adults use these complimentary therapies. According to the USA Commission for Alternative and Complimentary Medicines, people spent $17 billion on these remedies in 2000. The global market for herbal medicines is currently $60 billion annually and is growing.

People want to have healthy lifestyles, but they find it difficult to establish one. They want to eat healthy, but they don't know how. They believe exercise is important, but they don't know what to do, or they are not motivated to exercise. They think nutritional supplements are worthwhile, but are confused by conflicting information.

Therefore, chiropractors who have a complete system of products and services in place for their patients will greatly enhance their healing abilities and find that patients respond better—which is what our TrueChiro Health Management System is designed to do—to aid the doctor in a formula for diagnosis and treatment, nutritional advice and proper supplementation, plus corrective care exercises and motivation.

The rate of chronic degenerative disease in the U.S. continues to rise. One out of every two people dies from (easily prevented and treated) heart disease, which was virtually unknown less than one hundred years ago. One out of every three people dies from cancer. Diabetes is becoming an epidemic. And Alzheimer's disease currently impacts about five million people a year.

The number three cause of death in the U.S., as reported in the *Journal of the American Medical Association (JAMA)*, is doctors. Three years ago, a major national study found prescription errors, surgical complications, infections, and other medical mistakes killed 24,000 Canadians annually. (*Northern News*, November 30, 2007). Is it any wonder that people are leaving their doctors' offices still searching for answers?

Diseases that only a short time ago were thought to be part of the aging process are now found in young children. Twenty years ago, about 2 percent of all cases of new onset diabetes (Type II) were in people between nine and nineteen years old. Today, this age group accounts for about 30 to 50 percent. Likewise, heart disease, arthritis, and cancer are no longer just for the aged.

Even though there are thousands of books on diet and exercise, one in fifty adults is more than one hundred pounds overweight and two out of every three adults and one out of every five children are overweight. Many schools have been forced to obtain new scales that can measure 350 pounds and higher to monitor the weight of their students.

Ironically, while people in general are becoming sicker, we are in the midst of a health information overload. The airways and Internet provide vast amounts of information on hundreds of diets and supplements—but the sheer enormity brings confusion instead of clarity.

The TrueChiro Health Management Program we have designed incorporates the best diagnostic aspects of several natural therapies. It is not enough to only eat healthy. It is absolutely critical to customize your diet to your ever-changing needs. It is not enough to only exercise. Exercise must be done properly and, like your diet, must be customized to your specific needs. The TrueChiro Health Management Program teaches you how to eat right and make healthy food choices, and it will give you a better grasp of these principles while guiding you to a healthier life.

In order to achieve total health, you must take action. And to take action, you must have faith in the right system. Having faith in the wrong product or system will only produce disappointment. To gain total health you must start to think right and, as I tell my patients, you have to:

- get adjusted to think right
- get proper nutrients to think right
- get exercise to think right

Without movement, proper nerve flow, and good nutrition you lose life. If you think eating right, exercising, and getting adjusted seems daunting and a lot of work, don't worry. It takes no more energy to manage than the life of illness and fatigue you may have right now.

Actually it is not that hard to be healthy. You just have to make the right choices. You have to change your mind and put more energy into the direction you want to go rather than the direction you don't want to go.

The formula for change is when the desire for change is greater than the resistance to change. If you are ready to make a healthy change, then this is the program for you. If you want to continue to be sick and tired, then the choice is easy—don't change a thing!

On October 2, 2007, the Milken Institute released a report that stated the "annual economic impact of chronic disease on the U.S. economy is one trillion dollars." It also said that this could balloon to nearly six trillion dollars by the middle of the century.

Yet, the news is not entirely grim because much of this cost is *avoidable*. In every community of our country, people are suffering from *preventable* chronic diseases. What they need is education and guidance—and doctors of chiropractic must seize this opportunity to educate and provide TrueChiro Health Management to their patients.

According to the study, seven chronic diseases—cancer, diabetes, hypertension, stroke, heart disease, pulmonary condition, and mental illness—have a total impact on the economy of $1.3 trillion annually. Of this amount, $1.1 trillion represents the cost of lost productivity.

By investing in our health, with moderate improvements in prevention and early intervention, such as reducing the rate of obesity, the savings to the economy would be enormous.

This study is the first of its kind to estimate the *avoidable* costs if a serious effort were made to improve Americans' health. Assuming modest improvements in preventing and treating disease, Milken Institute researchers have determined that by 2023 the nation could avoid forty million cases of chronic disease and reduce the economic impact by 27 percent, or $1.1 trillion, annually. They also reported that the most important factor is obesity. If obesity rates declined, it could lead to $60 billion less in treatment costs and $254 billion in increased productivity.

This study is a call to action. It is time for people (and medical practitioners) to change how they view health. Making positive, healthier changes in one area of your life will lead to positive changes in other areas. When you choose to put proper nutrients into your body, you will begin to think and feel better. When you remove nervous system interference and allow proper nerve flow, your body becomes alive. When you begin to exercise, you expend and create new energy. When you change all areas at the same time, the results are positively life transforming.

You were born to be healthy, so if you are not experiencing total health, something is interfering. Is it your attitude, your diet, your exercise program, your sleep routine, and/or spinal misalignments blocking nerve transmission?

### DID YOU KNOW THAT:

- a positive attitude can improve your immune system?
- a proper meal plan can make you feel better about yourself?
- exercise can help with your social relationships?
- getting enough sleep can improve your chances of success?
- regular adjustments help in all areas of your life?

It is important to understand the relationship between your thoughts and your health in order to recognize how your thoughts have been running your life. This is where the TrueChiro Health Management Program is helpful. It will show you how to think differently and provide you with the principles and technique for doing so.

The definition of *health* is "a state of optimal physical, mental, and social well-being." It is not merely the absence of disease and infirmity. In other words, just because you don't have a disease or sickness doesn't necessarily mean you are healthy.

Total health is an optimally functioning state of mind, body, and spirit that allows for repair and regeneration of the body's cells, tissues, and organ systems at all times. Thus, disease is "any deviation or interruption of the normal structure or function of any part, organ, or system of the body and is manifested by a characteristic set of symptoms and signs and whose cause and prognosis may be known or unknown."

What, then, causes this deviation and how is it transmitted to cause disease?

Your body wants to be in a balanced state, also known as *homeostasis*. You have both internal and external environmental irritation that travels via the nervous system, trying to cause an imbalance in homeostasis. This irritation may be mechanical, chemical, or psychological and the determining factor in the cause of disease occurs when the irritation is greater than the body's resistance. If your body adapts or overcomes the irritation, there is health. However, every irritation that your nervous system comes in contact with adds to the irritant side and results in a relative decrease on the resistance side. This may go on until the limit is reached and adaptation can no longer occur, and disease is the result.

Note: if your nervous system is overloaded, your body is

# HOMEOSTASIS

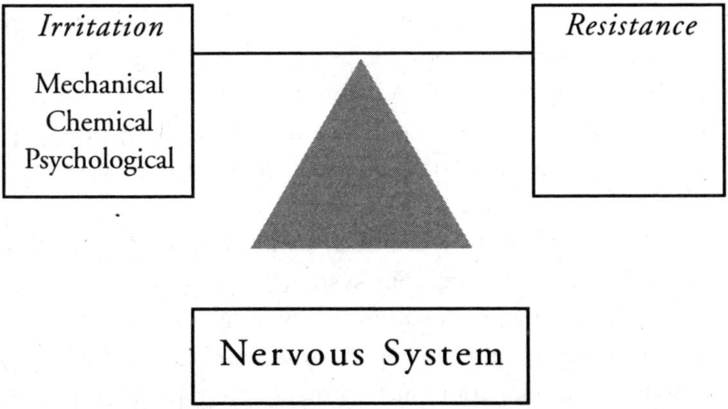


## Sickness

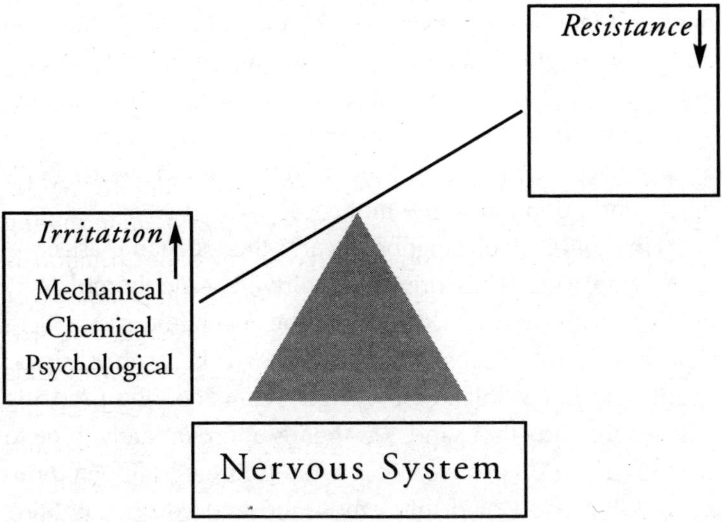

unable to adapt and sickness is present; therefore, in order to be healthy and balanced you must keep your nervous system free of interference and irritations.

First, your body must be free of nerve interference; second, you need the proper fuel; third, a strong body; and fourth, the right attitude. A combination of these elements will keep your cellular machinery running properly and help you produce the materials needed for repairing, replacing, and making all bodily fluids and structures. This remarkable process is directed by your body's inborn intelligence, also known as the central nervous system.

Let's pretend you are getting ready to take a long road trip with your family and you notice that your car isn't running smoothly. You take your car to a mechanic and, after a complete inspection, he says you need a new computer, the engine is going, and the frame has a serious defect in it.

You look at him and say, "How could this be? I have been driving this car for eight years and it has never given me a problem before. I have never had to put a penny into it. As a matter-of-fact, I have never even changed the oil!" Then you add, "My neighbor is constantly bringing in his car. He gets his car inspected and maintained three or four times a year. You know what they say, once you bring your car in, you always have to bring it in. I just don't see the benefit . . . it's costly and I don't have the time."

"How old is your neighbor's car?" the mechanic asks.

You answer, "He's driving a thirty-year-old bomb! Why would anyone want to do that?" The mechanic says, "Let's look at the overall cost. Thirty years ago, he probably paid twenty thousand dollars for it. Eight years ago, you probably paid about thirty thousand. He spends approximately three to five hundred dollars a year, for a total of nine to fifteen thousand dollars. You paid thirty thousand and you put nothing into maintenance, which means you will need three cars in thirty years, for a total of ninety to one hundred thousand dollars. That is a difference of eighty-five to ninety-one thousand dollars! Would you like to save that kind of money? Do you see how maintenance can keep a car running well and save you money?"

"Yes, but I still don't have the time!"

"Well, I can't help you there. All I can tell you is everyone gets twenty-four hours in a day. I see some very busy people in town bringing their cars in for maintenance on a regular basis. So, that tells me it's about priorities. Make regular maintenance a priority and you will save money—plus have a well running piece of machinery that won't let you down."

The choices you make have consequences. If you choose to neglect your car, it will break down. If you choose to neglect your body, it will also let you down.

Unfortunately, we live in a society where crisis motivates people to change. It takes cancer, a heart attack, or the death of a close friend for most of us to start thinking about how precious our health is. This is called a *paradoxical health approach*, where poor health inspires us to be well. It is an approach that may leave you in the hospital bed or nursing home instead of outside enjoying an active healthy lifestyle.

Wouldn't it be better if you chose to change now, because you wanted to and not later because you had to?

If you focus on the quality of life you want, the changes will be easier. Picture in your mind where you will be in one, two, and five years. What is your perfect day like? How are you mentally? How are you physically? How are you socially? Picture what you want to change in your life today and start the process towards that life. Change happens one choice at a time. Making better choices today will impact the level of your health in the future.

By taking control of your own health, you begin what is called *self-care*. It is what you do to keep yourself functioning at your highest level, which nobody else can do for you. Self-care is about the choices you make every day. It is about being responsible for your health, which includes eating the right foods, getting the proper amount of exercise, and taking care of your supporting structure, i.e., your spine.

Most people struggle with positive change because they think it is hard or they don't have time. Taking care of yourself isn't hard. What is difficult is changing your everyday pattern from a destructive or complacent one to a constructive or productive one. Remember change is easy, thinking about change is hard.

When you take good care of yourself, you will have more energy. You will need less sleep and, therefore, you will have more time. If taking care of yourself has not been the norm, now is the time to start, before a crisis occurs. And, realize, that before you can effectively take care of someone else, you must first take care of yourself.

One healthy choice leads to another. Feeling great after you eat leads to other healthy food choices. Feeling the energy flow through your body after an adjustment makes you more aware of what is occurring in your body.

Taking good care of yourself will keep your immune system strong so that your resistance to infection remains high. Have you ever noticed that healthy people are less likely to get sick or when they do get sick they don't seem to be affected as bad? Sick people seem to attract sickness. That is because their bodies are good hosts for disease; their resistance is low. By keeping yourself healthy with good self-care, you are attracting a quality life.

To keep yourself functioning at your best you must utilize the knowledge and skill of a trained health professional. This is the proactive way and it is the type of healthcare you can not provide for yourself.

It is important to keep your body in a state of homeostasis. To do this, you must make sure your nervous system is free of interference, your stress level is at a minimum, you eat a healthy diet, and you have a good exercise plan. Following a TrueChiro Health Management System will keep you in the best health of your life.

Healthcare is about keeping your mind, body, and spirit strong. You must understand that your body is designed to be healthy. Disease is not normal and you need to stop thinking of disease as part of the aging process. Every day I have people say to me, "I just came back from the doctor and he says I have degenerative joint disease (osteoarthritis) in my hip, knee, spine, etc. He says nothing can be done; it's just a normal part of aging. Then he gave me a prescription."

I say, "Oh, really? Let's have a look at your x-rays." I point to the degeneration on the right hip, fourth and fifth lumbar, etc. And then I find a healthy joint and ask them, "Is this joint the same age as the unhealthy one?"

Their answer is always yes. "So, it's not a part of the aging process, then," I say.

I explain that I have seen x-rays of older people who don't have much degeneration. Therefore this degeneration is due to the joint being misaligned for a long period of time.

You see, disease is a process; you don't just wake up one morning and have osteoarthritis, heart disease, or cancer. You may wake up one morning with a symptom; but the disease process has been occurring over time. Just like health is a process, so is disease.

You have a choice on the process and direction you want to take. Excellent healthcare with great self-care will keep your body functioning at its optimum.

A health-care team should consist of knowledgeable providers who see your health with a multifaceted approach, and/or have a TrueChiro Health Management System in place. This system should be the foundation of health. Every healthy choice you make adds to your pyramid of health—but remember, it is this strong foundation that you build upon. Building on a weak foundation only results in a collapse of your health.

Your primary health foundation should consist of four areas:

**Chiropractic**—to keep your spine and nervous system healthy

**Nutrition**—for a healthy diet and proper supplementation

**Exercise**—to keep your body in shape

**Psychological**—to develop the right frame of mind for life events

Disease and dysfunction are caused by irritation of the nervous system. The irritation can be physical/mechanical,

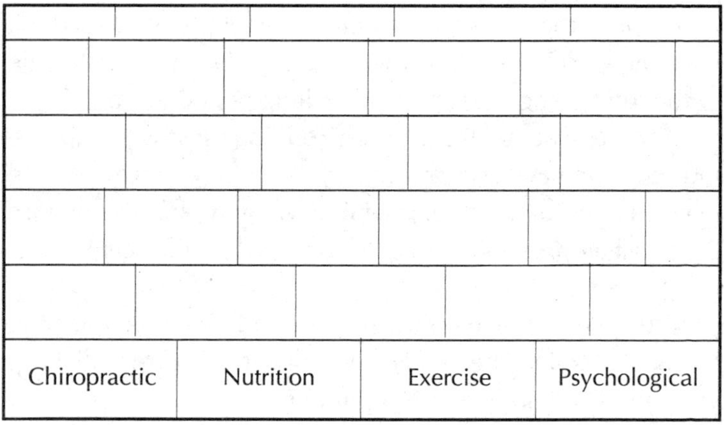

chemical, or psychological. The irritations of the nervous system may result in an upset of the body's homeostasis and result in disease.

Various treatments are available to restore your health: an adjustment of the spine to keep your nervous system healthy and/or to reset it; a fascial technique to release the kinetic chain; massage therapy, to deal with muscular imbalances and help deal with stress; personal trainer for conditioning and corrective exercises; a change of diet and or supplementation to deal with chemical imbalances; or an attitude adjustment to deal with your psyche.

Certain aspects will require daily attention, while other areas need not be so frequent. It's sort of like your dental care, i.e., brushing your teeth daily is necessary whereas seeing your dentist daily is not.

Developing good health habits will ensure that your mind, body, and spirit function at their fullest potential. The more you neglect your self-care and healthcare, the more frequently you will be visiting a crisis-care team, which is where you go to recover from an injury or illness and it may require

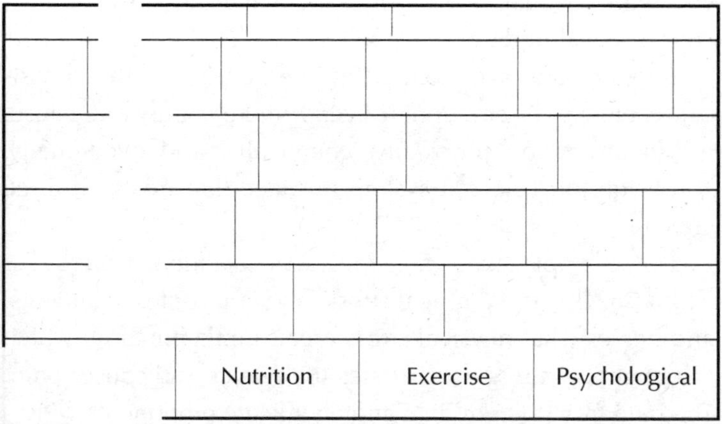

the support of medications, surgery, and/or hospitalization. Crisis management is expensive and does not guarantee long-term quality of life. At some point in your life you may need crisis care. However, being as healthy as possible will ensure a speedier recovery.

The best approach begins by accepting responsibility for your own health. This means staying informed; making changes in your daily life (such as diet, exercise, attitude, and chiropractic care); maintaining, supporting, and building on your health foundation; and, finally, having in place the best doctors and a TrueChiro Health Management System. Your day-to-day health choices will strengthen your entire being, which is your best ally to remain healthy as you age and postpone any crisis for as long as possible.

Start by looking at your posture. Are you standing straight or do you slouch? Are you working toward a healthy heart? Are you making your mind and body stronger?

Everything begins with your thoughts. Your thoughts are who you are; they are your experiences of being. You decide what ideas to accept and which ones to reject. You decide what to think and what to feel. When these decisions leave you with residual stress, you experience the stress as if in your physical body.

Stress creates symptoms. The question is, are they physical, chemical, or emotional? Even if there is only one cause, it can affect you physically, chemically, and emotionally. Thus, you must have a system in place that treats all three areas.

For example, you are in a car accident and suffer whiplash. That is a physical stress to your muscles, ligaments, and nerves. That physical stress creates inflammation, which is a chemical stress that irritates the nerves and causes pain. The pain from the physical and chemical components causes emotional stress, resulting in a psychological factor. This can lead to developing patterns in your body.

Have you ever wondered why stress affects everyone differently? Why does an emotional stress affect one person in the lower back while causing someone else to suffer from heart or stomach ailments? People come into my office with chronic subluxations in the same places all the time. When I ask them what they did to cause this, they might say, "I didn't do anything. I had a funeral to go to and I drove five hours, ate in restaurants, and slept in a hotel."

All this stress—physical from driving in one position for too long and sleeping in a different bed, emotional from the driving and the death, and chemical from eating restaurant food—enters the conscious and subconscious mind, gets processed, and travels down the nervous system affecting the spine, muscles, and organs. Now, enter this stress into an already unhealthy spine and nervous system and you have an overload on the body that will result in signs and symptoms affecting the muscles, organs, and decreased immune system; headaches, fatigue . . . and the list goes on and on.

What can you do?

1. Don't wait for a crisis to motivate you to better health. Remember your health is your responsibility and your choice.

2. Start a self-care program and follow it daily. Here are some examples:

   a. Daily exercise for at least twenty minutes

   b. Restful sleep (six to eight hours)

   c. Drink plenty of water (at least eight to ten glasses)

   d. Proper nutrition (eating a balanced diet)

   e. Attitude (read, listen, and think positively)

3. Get a Health-Care Team in place. If you can, find a chiropractor with a TrueChiro Health Management System that identifies the areas you need treated, the different types of treatment, the nutritional and proper supplementation, and the corrective exercises for you. However, if you can't find a chiropractor with a TrueChiro Health Management System, then you should interview a chiropractor, naturopath, massage therapist, general practitioner, personal trainer, and a nutritionist.

4. Don't be afraid of change. Change is easy—thinking about change is hard. Make the changes you know you need to make. Don't think about it, take action.

5. Educate yourself. Become a student of good health.

6. Enjoy the journey. It is not about reaching your goals, it is about the journey; that is where you live, learn, and laugh. That is where your mind and body begin to feel and look younger.

Please understand that where you find yourself tomorrow is a result of the decisions and actions you take today. TrueChiro Health Management will help you discover what is right for you. To enjoy the best of times, follow the advice of this program and your doctor of chiropractic

You may contact Drs. Michel and Angel Dupuis at:

213 Whitewood Avenue, Norland Building
New Liskeard, Ontario P0J 1K0
Box 1479
Email: drmichel@gooddaychiropractic.com
www.TrueChiroHealth.com

# 6.

# Think Outside the Box

## Dr. Richard Tapper

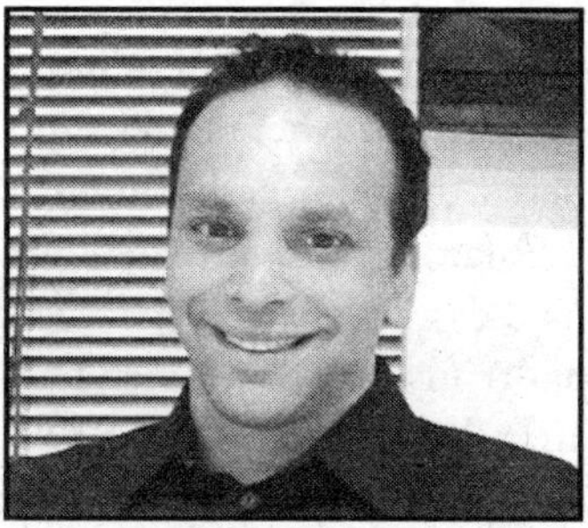

**Dr. Richard Tapper** graduated from the University of Winnipeg in 1998 with a Bachelor of Science degree. He attended Southern California University of Health Sciences where he completed his Doctorate in Chiropractic in 2002.

Dr. Tapper opened his first practice in Winnipeg in 2003. He has since opened two other clinics in Gimli and Niverville. In May 2004, he was awarded Chiropractor of the Month by the international organization Chiropractic Leadership Alliance, in recognition of his extraordinary vision and his passion for excellence. Dr. Tapper was also the British Columbia Lions' Chiropractor for the 2004 and 2006 Grey Cups.

An international speaker, Dr. Tapper has presented seminars on healthy living and personal development and achievement to numerous companies, including RBC, Pattison Signs, City Mix, B'nai B'rith, and DCS in Edmonton, Alberta. He has trained under Bob Proctor and Dr. John Demartini, teachers from the popular movie and bestselling book *The Secret.*

Dr. Tapper continues to strive for excellence and believes that a healthy mind and a healthy spine lead to a healthy life. His mission is to inspire people to reach their full potential in mind, body, and spirit.

My story starts in the north end of Winnipeg, Manitoba, in a working class neighborhood where I grew up. The north end of Winnipeg is considered the poor end of town. My life, however, was the opposite. My family was extremely wealthy in love and support. My parents, Leya and Bernie, did everything they could to nurture and support my sister and me. They worked hard to give us the things that they were unable to have as children.

Even though we could barely afford it, my parents sent me to a private school and summer camp every year. Through my parents' hard work and determination I learned the meaning of the words *inspired* and *inspiration.* They were my inspiration; they showed me that as long as you put your mind and your heart into something, anything can be accomplished.

Upon finishing high school, my goal was simple: attend university, get a Bachelor of Science degree, and then head off to chiropractic school. Up until that point, I had never been to a chiropractor but something was calling me into the profession.

I graduated from the University of Winnipeg and attended chiropractic school in Southern California. Chiropractic school changed the course of my life forever. I forged amazing relationships that still exist today; and, more importantly, I also learned the power of the body and how chiropractic truly saves lives. I did not learn this only in my classes; I learned it by visiting the offices of many of the most powerful chiropractors in the United States. These amazing doctors showed me that miracles can be everyday occurrences and they showed me the power that makes the body heal itself.

I learned that chiropractic is not only about back pain and neck pain; rather it is about allowing the body to heal the way it was intended, from above down, inside and out.

My excitement continued to grow and when I graduated from chiropractic school in December 2002, I knew I wanted to see this amazing healing power firsthand.

While my first clinic was being built, I set up a clinic in a homeless shelter. I was doing what I was taught to do: give, give, and keep on giving. People lined up every day to get adjusted. The first experience I had with the power of chiropractic was when one gentleman who had such a strong belief in what I did removed his wife from the hospital and carried her into my makeshift office. As he set her on the exam table, he said, "They are killing my wife. Please, you must help her."

I was twenty-six years old and fresh out of chiropractic school. I did what I knew—I examined her spine for subluxations and adjusted the segments that needed to be adjusted. The adjustment released such a power in her body that as soon as it was delivered her eyes popped open and she muttered, "Thank you." We all started to cry and I knew I had reached my calling. I had experienced the amazing power of the adjustment and the fantastic ability of the human body to heal on its own.

**A** zoo in Colorado decided to build one of the world's best polar bear reserves. In anticipation of the opening, a polar bear cub was purchased. While the reserve was being built, the cub was kept in a cage. While in the cage, the bear could only take two steps to the left and two steps to the right.

The project, which was supposed to only take one year, ended up taking nine years to complete! By this time, the cub was a fully grown polar bear.

The big day arrived and the bear was set to be released into the great reserve. The cage was placed in the middle of the compound and the bear was set free. To the shock of everyone, the bear would only take two steps to the left and two steps to the right. In its mind, it was still inside the box.

Likewise, when it comes to health, many people are stuck in a box where they think good health is based on luck and chance. In fact, health is based on the decisions you make. You have the ability to change your health forever once you start thinking outside the box.

Chiropractic is one of the most misunderstood and controversial professions. Being a chiropractor has helped me understand what Christopher Columbus must have gone through when he was trying to convince people that the world was round.

When it comes to health, we live in a flat world today; one dominated by dogma, habit, and backward thinking. If I asked ten different people the definition of *health*, I would get ten different answers.

Society trusts a health-care system that is destroying more lives than it saves. Don't get me wrong, the practice of medicine is great *when used for the correct purpose*.

Medicine is intended to be used for crisis and trauma situations only. If you are walking down the street and a car hits you, do you want to be in my office? Of course not. Go to a hospital where they can help you. In terms of crisis and trauma, a hospital is the best place to be. Everything else, though, has developed into sick care, i.e., there is little healthcare to be delivered.

Every year, medicine is listed as one of the five leading causes of death. How can it be that a system that is supposed to save people is actually killing hundreds of thousands in North America each year? The reason is money. Medical doctors have lost control of their own system, which is now being run by the pharmaceutical industry. And, this industry has one goal: to make money. It is an industry dominated by greed and power.

How many lives are lost annually to an industry that is experimenting with your health and your trust? How many drugs are pulled off the market each year because of the damage they cause? It is time to take back what is truly yours: your health.

What is the definition of *health*? Most say health is about feeling good. If this is the definition you live by, your health could be in danger.

Most symptoms do not show up until the body is functioning at 60 percent or less. If you are functioning at 65 percent you are definitely not healthy—but you may feel great. It is like having a cavity in your tooth, i.e., you won't know it is there until it is too late. Once you feel the cavity, the dentist either must fill it or pull the tooth. The cavity did not happen overnight, even though the pain may have come on suddenly.

This also happens with your health. It may take years and years for you to feel a symptom—even though disease has been ravaging your body for a long time. For most people, their first sign of heart disease is an actual heart attack; and by then it is often too late. Heart disease has been forming in the body for years, yet the person was unaware.

If the definition of *health* is not "feeling good," what is it? The true definition of *health* is having a body, mind, and spirit functioning at 100 percent. How do you know if your body is functioning at 100 percent?

Generally, people believe that a medical doctor can determine if their body is functioning at 100 percent by performing various tests. However, this belief can be dangerous to your health because most medical tests will show you when you *have* the disease but oftentimes nothing detrimental shows up on tests when you are actually *developing* the disease. In other words, tests for cancer and heart disease don't warn you that you are developing a disease.

Realize though, heart disease and cancer do not suddenly appear; it takes years for these conditions to develop, even if only months before a test was negative and now it happens to be positive.

Again I ask: how do you know if your body is functioning at full potential? To answer this question, you must first understand how the human body works and what controls it.

Your brain is the master control system; it controls all bodily functions and systems. It is your hard drive. Attached to the brain is the spinal cord, and coming off this cord are nerves. These nerves transmit messages sent by the brain, down the spinal cord, and exit through the spine to every structure and cell in your body.

Each nerve controls a different part of your body. There are nerves that make your heart beat; your lungs contract; your knees, toes, and ankles move, etc.

When your brain is able to send its messages effectively down the spinal cord to the nerves, and the nerves are able to get the information to their particular destinations, then your body can heal and function to the best of its ability. Your spine protects your brain stem and spinal cord, and allows nerves to exit from the spinal cord. It is made up of seven bones in the neck, twelve in the middle back, and five in the lower back. When your spine is in the correct alignment, these nerves are able to flow freely from the brain to the rest of your body and back again.

However, when your spine shifts out of its normal position, it will put tremendous pressure on the brain stem and will pinch and damage the spinal cord and nerves. This pinching is called a *subluxation*. A subluxation can be defined as a bone out of place in your spine that pinches and chokes off nerves.

A subluxation is dangerous because it disrupts nerve communication. Consider this: if someone was to cut the nerve to your tooth, your tooth would die. Imagine if you had a bone out of place that was pinching the nerve going to your stomach. There would be less nerve flow to the stomach, which means the stomach would not be able to perform as required, and eventually the stomach is going to get sick and die. It's just like your tooth; your stomach is moving towards a slow death without you knowing it. Subluxations can cause pain but, more importantly, they destroy your body, and cause disease and early death. The only professionals trained to detect and correct subluxations are chiropractors.

When was the last time you or your children were checked for subluxation? When was the last time your spine was x-rayed? For most people, the answer is never. The only time that most people seek out chiropractic care is when they are in pain.

As you now know, pain is when your body is functioning at 60 percent or less—which is not the best way to deal with your most important asset, your health.

Chiropractic was never meant for just back and neck pain. Dr. D. D. Palmer, the founder of chiropractic, discovered and promoted chiropractic as a method of care to allow the body to heal and function to the best of its ability.

If you break your arm, your body heals it. If you cut yourself, your body heals it. Every day your body produces cancer cells and every day your body fights them off through your immune system that is controlled by your brain.

If the messages (nerves) from your brain are blocked, eventually your body will not be able to fight off disease and your health will deteriorate. Your body has the greatest pharmacy, healing power, and stitching system in the universe; however, if this healing power from your brain is blocked, I guarantee your body will go into a state of dis-ease.

There are three ways your body forms these devastating and life-threatening subluxations. The first is physical stress. Physical stress includes car accidents, falls, trauma at birth, sitting at a computer all day, poor posture, and heavy labor. The second is chemical stress, which includes drugs and poor food that you ingest. If you swallow a bottle of aspirin, you will die. By taking one aspirin every day you are killing yourself slowly. Drugs are not meant to be taken daily for the rest of your life. They are meant to be temporary solutions, until the cause can be found. And, once the cause is determined, it's time to do something to change.

North Americans have the poorest eating habits in the world. They are constantly feeding their bodies processed foods, large amounts of sugar and sodium, and too much fast food. If you had a Porsche you would likely put the best oil and gas in it. Think of your body as a Porsche; always put the best materials into it. Think of quality healthy food as high-octane fuel for your body. This will allow it to run best.

The third cause of subluxations is emotional stress, which can be as or more devastating to your body than chemical and physical stress combined.

The goal of chiropractic is simple; yet so vital: find subluxations and correct them. Chiropractors detect subluxations through x-rays, special computer technology, and physical exams. Once subluxations are detected, the goal is simple: restore the correct alignment in the spine and allow the body to heal and function at its best.

If there is a subluxation affecting the nerve going to the heart, the heart will not function correctly. Changes that can occur include elevated blood pressure, chest pain, etc. These are signals the body sends to tell the individual that there is a problem. How do most people react to these signs? Usually they try to eliminate the signal and not the cause, which is why so many people are taking blood pressure medication.

A recent study determined that spinal adjustments of subluxations of the upper part of the cervical spine (neck) are as effective, if not more effective, in regulating blood pressure. "Anatomical abnormalities of the cervical spine at the level of the Atlas vertebra are associated with relative ischemia of the brainstem circulation and increased blood pressure (BP). Manual correction of this mal-alignment has been associated with reduced arterial pressure. This pilot study tests the hypothesis that correcting mal-alignment of the Atlas vertebra reduces and maintains a lower BP. Using a double blind, placebo-controlled design at a single center, 50 drug naïve (n=26) or washed out (n=24) patients with Stage 1 hypertension were randomized to receive a National Upper Cervical Chiropractic (NUCCA) procedure or a sham procedure. Patients received no antihypertensive meds during the 8-week study duration. The primary end point was changed in systolic and diastolic BP comparing baseline and week 8, with a 90% power to detect an 8/5 mm Hg difference at week 8 over the placebo group."[1]

Simply trying to eliminate symptoms is like a fireman disconnecting the alarm rather than focusing on putting out the fire. The alarm is a signal that there is a fire. Likewise, symptoms are your body's way of telling you that there is a fire inside you. Do not eliminate the alarm; take out the fire.

In the last ten years, North American pharmaceutical companies have done more research on heart disease, cancer, and stroke than ever before. Has this decreased the number of patients afflicted by these terrible diseases? No. In actuality, the opposite is happening. The number of people afflicted has increased significantly.

How can this be? No drug can remove pressure off a nerve to free up communication. If all we do is take care of symptoms, people will continue to get sicker and sicker.

Most people develop subluxations the day they are born. A doctor pulling on a baby's neck can cause the spinal bone at the top of the neck to misalign and put major pressure on these nerves, which is why it is important to get newborns checked as soon as possible. If the subluxation is found right away and corrected the body will be able to heal and function properly.

Common signs and symptoms of spinal subluxation in babies include recurrent ear infections, colic, ADD, stomach issues, and bed wetting.

Disease is a body's way of showing us that it is unable to handle things internally.

A lot of people believe that illness is the result of germs. I hate to break it to you—but germs are everywhere.

How can one hundred people walk into a room and eighty stay healthy while twenty get sick? Especially since all of them were exposed to the same germs.

The reason is that eighty people had a strong immune system and were able to combat the germs, while the others had a weakened immune system.

What controls the immune system? The brain and nervous system. Therefore, when your spine is lined up correctly your brain is able to communicate with your body and your body can fight almost everything off.

What is the value of a strong immune system? When your immune system is not working, your body will succumb to germs that people with strong immune systems can easily fight off. Dr. Fred Barge illustrated the point in this way. He likened it to rats in a dump. If you remove the rats in a dump, a few weeks later they will return. However, if you take away the dump, the rats have no where to live. Likewise, if your body has a healthy environment, disease is unable to manifest.

By changing the environment inside of your body, you are changing the health of your body. Changing the internal environment is done through removing subluxations and allowing your brain and body to connect so your body can function as close to 100 percent as possible. Such a simple concept; yet simplicity is hard for many people to accept.

The symptoms and conditions that patients present with in my office never cease to amaze me. From infertility, to Chrohn's disease, fibromyalgia, ADD, cancer, heart disease, etc. it all has been seen—and most have been helped tremendously with chiropractic care.

The one concept that needs to be understood is that a chiropractor *facilitates* healing by correcting subluxations; it is *your body* that does the healing. A chiropractor removes the subluxation that is interfering with the nervous system and preventing your body from healing. Once the interference is removed, your body can heal the way it was intended.

My mother started getting adjusted as soon as I opened my first clinic. At the time, she was on twelve different medications, including blood pressure pills, diabetic pills, anti-inflammatory medication, and water pills. Today, she is off every single one of these medications. She is healthier at the age of sixty-two than she was at the age of forty-five.

Her healthy transformation did not happen overnight. It took almost four years for her body to heal. Her spine will never be fully corrected; but the interference is being removed twice a week so that my mother can lead a much more active and fulfilled life. If you ask her the value of getting adjusted, she will tell you it saved her life.

And that is the essence of chiropractic: saving lives. It is about allowing people to have an amazing quality of life. It allows people to express health to the best of their ability.

Once the spine is corrected, it needs to be maintained. My patients want to maintain their spines for the rest of their lives.

We teach the chiropractic lifestyle to all our patients. This includes checking their spines on a regular basis and eliminating the stresses that cause life-devastating subluxations.

Exercise is one of the most important things you can do for your body. Your body was meant to move. It was not meant to sit at a desk all day or be on a couch for hours while ingesting terrible food and watching TV.

The work many people perform and the computers they sit at cause their spines to deteriorate at a much faster rate compared to their ancestors. That said, if your spine is not properly aligned, it may be more dangerous to exercise, which is why so many professional athletes receive regular chiropractic care.

At a recent seminar, I heard New York Yankee Johnny Damon and football players Barry Larkin and Duane Clemmons share the importance of chiropractic in their personal and professional lives.

If you exercise on a bad spine, do you think it will get better or worse? The answer, of course, is worse. That is why people who want active and healthy lifestyles include chiropractic in their routines.

We teach good nutrition. One of the best illustrations of the body telling you that you are killing it with poor food is heartburn. However, instead of changing the food eaten, which is creating significant stress on the body, people decide to take heartburn medication that allows them to eat unhealthy food without feeling the heartburn. Does this make sense to you?

One of the most significant stresses that must be dealt with is emotional stress. The way you think and the emotions you feel can have a major effect on your nervous system and ultimately on the health of your body and the quality of your life. In the book *Hidden Messages in Water*, Professor Masuru Emoto describes research whereby he placed water in different containers, wrote specific words on the bottles, and subjected the water molecules to different sounds, music, or statements. He then froze the water and analyzed the ice crystals under a microscope. The first test group had positive words sprinkled all over the bottles; such as *love, thank you*, and *fantastic*. In the positive group, the crystals were well formed and beautiful. Emoto took another set of bottles and wrote words such as *hate, killer*, and *murder* on them. He placed these crystals under the same microscope and discovered malformed, visually unappealing, and ugly crystals. Emoto repeated these experiments over ten years and came up with the same results over and over again. The most beautiful, symmetrical, and organized crystals were formed when the water was subjected to positive, enriching, and supportive words.[2]

How is this important to your health and healing? A large percentage of your body is made up of water molecules; researchers say as much as 70 to 90 percent of the human body, depending on age and other factors. The words you speak to yourself and others are important because they can have a major impact on your health. Most obvious is that being in a state of gratitude will allow you to be in the best of health and allow your beauty to shine through.

Unfortunately, most people do not treat themselves like this. They oftentimes use negative and nasty words. If I spoke to most people the way they talk to themselves, they would dislike me in five minutes.

Negative thoughts have been shown to put a great deal of stress on the spine and nervous system. By constantly being in a state of worry and panic, your posture is affected; there are obvious changes in your physiology and, therefore, changes in your health.

By speaking to yourself and others with loving and caring words you will positively impact your health. To experience dramatic changes in your emotional well-being, all it takes are positive affirmations every day and spending five to ten minutes in gratitude for what you have and for what you are able to give.

Life was meant to be enjoyed and abundant; yet so many people live either in future fear or past guilt. Once you learn how to be present in the moment, the stresses of the past and the fear of the future will dissolve. It only requires a little discipline and planning.

It is said that those who fail to plan, are ultimately planning to fail. The majority spend more time planning a vacation than planning their lives. The biggest reason: most were never taught the importance of goal setting, making plans, and following through. When a plan is set, emotional stress melts away. When emotional stress is decreased to a minimum, the spine has a greater chance of being subluxation free. A subluxation-free life is an amazing life.

Ask any elderly person what the most important thing in his life is and he will say his health.

What is your health worth? How do you know you are healthy? Who do you trust to guide and serve you to care for your health?

If you see a physician and receive drugs every time you are sick, you are making a grave error. Can you trust a system that is killing so many people? Doesn't it make more sense to create a lifestyle that brings you closer to health, rather than making decisions that pull you away? Are you preventing illness from happening to you and your children or are you managing illnesses as they occur?

In my opinion, health is priceless.

Consider the mother who came into my office because her son could only go to the bathroom once a month. This child had seen every specialist and taken every concoction imaginable. After a thorough chiropractic examination, I found a severe subluxation in the boy's lower spine. After a month of getting adjusted, he was able to go to the bathroom daily.

Is that a miracle? No. That is what occurs when the body functions without nerve interference.

What value do you think this child and his mother place on chiropractic; a child who can now play with his friends, go to sleepovers, and not worry about all the toxins that were accumulating in his body? You are right; to that parent and child the chiropractic experience and reward are priceless.

Not only is the child under our care, so is the entire family. The mother told me, "My family has never been happier in its life."

Such experiences take place every day in my office.

None of our practice members under regular care has gotten cancer or heart disease, yet those diseases are the number one and number two killers in North America. Are people in my office just lucky—or are they truly healthy?

How long do you want your child to be healthy? For most parents, the answer is forever.

You owe it yourself, your children, and your children's children to be healthy. It is time to take control of your health. It is time to be a health manager instead of a disease manager.

Chiropractic is where the impossible becomes the possible, from within. The Latin term *lux* means light or energy, so *subluxation* means a condition of less light or less energy. By getting adjusted you are turning the power on and letting the light of who you are truly shine through.

B. J. Palmer, the developer of chiropractic, put it this way: "Do we have more faith in a knife or a spoonful of medicine than the power that animates the body?" Fortunately more people are starting to understand the truth about health and healing and are embarking on the wellness path—a path that includes the chiropractic lifestyle.

Two thousand years ago, in a small town outside of Jerusalem, there was a man who was considered to be a psychic. Some of the children decided to test the skills of this so-called wise man. They went to the man and asked him, "What are we holding behind our backs?"

The wise man thought and, while he was thinking, he saw a feather rise to the sky. The man said, "Well, kids. It seems as though you have a bird behind your back."

The children were in shock and decided to huddle up for a few minutes and then went back to the man. They asked him, "Is the bird dead or alive?"

The old man pondered for a few minutes. He realized if he said the bird was alive, they would certainly kill the bird. If he said the bird was dead, they would make him look like a fool. He finally answered, "Well, kids. The answer is in your hands."

His answer is reflective of how most people live their lives. The answer is always in your hands. You are where you are today because of the choices and decisions you made yesterday, last week, last month, etc. You will be where you are tomorrow based on the decisions you start making today.

The decision of health is an inside-out job, not an outside-in one. If you decide that your health and that of your children is a number one priority, then seeing a chiropractor is your best decision. If you aren't sure, all you have to do is ask people who decide to go through the chiropractic corrective care process and maintain it forever. For them, a chiropractic lifestyle for life has become a priority.

A healthy individual leads to a healthy family; and healthy families create healthy communities, cities, countries, and world.

Inside the word *health* is the word *heal* and inside your spine is how you heal; therefore, an aligned spine will always keep you healthy. A patient of mine said it best:

> "Chiropractic care cannot be defined by adjustments to my spine; instead it should be measured by the improvement in my quality of life."

Contact Dr. Richard Tapper at:

1-1325 Markham Road
Winnipeg, Manitoba, Canada R3t 4j6
Telephone: 204-275-5030.
Email: doctapper@hotmail.com

## References

1. G. Bakris, M. Dickholtz Sr., P. M. Meyer, G. Kravitz, E. Avery, M. Miller, J. Brown, C. Woodfield, and B. Bell. *Journal of Human Hypertension*, 2 March 2007.

2. Emoto, Masuru. *Hidden Messages in Water*, 2001.

# 7.

# Who is Responsible For Your Health?

Dr. D. J. LeDrew

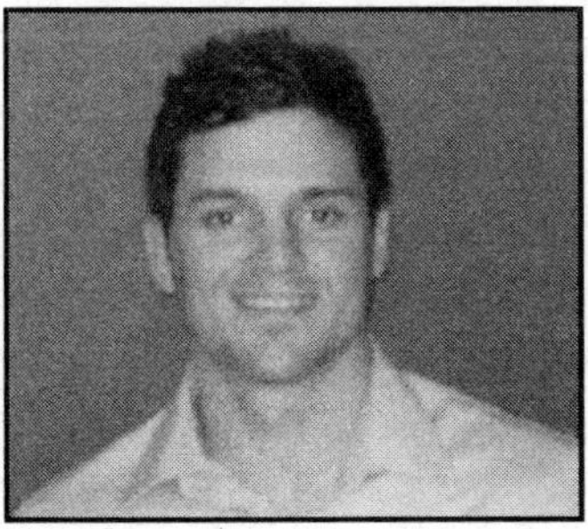

My chiropractic story begins when I was a child suffering from severe migraine headaches. After extensive testing and investigation within the conventional medical system—to no avail—my parents turned to another solution: chiropractic!

After one spinal adjustment, my life changed. For the first time in years, I had complete relief from debilitating migraines. From that point on, I was intrigued by chiropractic and began to ponder becoming a chiropractor.

I began my post-secondary studies at the University of Calgary (U of C), where I graduated with a bachelor's degree in kinesiology with an emphasis in mind sciences.

During my tenure at U of C, I wrestled for the varsity team

and learned the value of hard work by juggling my studies and athletic training.

In 2000, I was recognized as the University of Calgary Scholar Athlete of the Year, one of my proudest moments. I am grateful for the life lessons learned during my ten-year wrestling career. During those years, I was a five time national medallist and three time National Champion, representing Canada at many international competitions.

Although I was just reaching my prime in wrestling, I decided to move on to chiropractic and fulfill my mission of serving humanity instead of pursuing the Olympic dream.

I attended the Los Angeles College of Chiropractic because Southern California is a chiropractic mecca and has more schools and chiropractors than anywhere else in the world. I also figured I would get the best exposure—and, if I was going to study for another four years, why not do it in sunny California?

When I began classes in January 2001, I set the goal that I wanted to graduate at the top of my class. I felt if I didn't learn the material well enough, it would be a disservice to my future patients. I achieved that goal: I graduated as the valedictorian, summa cum laude, and was selected by the National Board of Chiropractic Examiners as the fee waiver recipient, which means they paid for my national board exam fee. While in chiropractic college, I also attended many weekend seminars to ensure that I was fully prepared for practice with the most current knowledge.

I began a solo practice in Calgary, Alberta, in January 2005; and still remain. I maintain one of the busiest family wellness chiropractic offices in the city, and contribute to the wrestling community where I am the team chiropractor for the Canadian National Wrestling Team working out of the Canadian National Sport Center at the University of Calgary.

I have a passion for ongoing learning and continue to expand my knowledge by attending regular post-graduate conferences to provide my patients with the most current chiropractic care.

It is a chilly winter afternoon in a Detroit suburb. In a hockey arena parents cheer and scream in support of the young boys who are giving their all on the ice. In an instant the arena goes silent. Every face is frozen in a state of complete shock.

"Somebody call 9-1-1!" the referee hollers, with a tremble in his voice.

A player lays on the ice, unable to move from the neck down, tears rolling down one side of his face. The boy looks up to find a familiar face of comfort in the crowd that surrounds him. "Coach, coach," he whimpers.

"Yes, I'm here," is the reply.

"What happened? I went into the corner to get the puck and . . . and I didn't do anything wrong . . . I looked behind me . . . no one was there," the boy stutters.

"He came out of the penalty box after you looked; you couldn't have seen him," the coach mumbles.

"Mom!" he cries out.

"Yes, sweetie. I'm here. It's going to be okay." She is crying and has a blank look on her face.

"Mommy, I can't feel my legs or my arms. I'm scared," the boy says.

"I know, honey. But don't worry. You'll be okay. Just lay still, okay? The ambulance is almost here," she says, as she frantically looks over both shoulders as if to reassure herself.

Over the next few hours, the boy gradually regains feeling in his legs, then his arms, until he is completely recovered. He is released from the hospital shortly thereafter with a collar on his neck and instructions to see his doctor when he returns home. Although the doctors said he'd never play contact sports again, the boy went back to playing hockey!

Prior to the accident, he experienced migraine headaches; they are now more frequent and severe. He spends days in a catatonic state in a dark room with a cold washcloth on his head.

Countless hours are spent in doctors' offices in search of the cause and a cure. The multiple diagnostic tests performed give no insight to the root of the migraines. The only solution is noxious medication that knocks him out, worse than the headaches. At least without the medication he would have a few normal days between migraines. He merely wants to be like every other boy his age and go to school or play hockey—but the migraines prevent this. He can't understand why he has to suffer so much; he just wants to be normal.

While watching him play hockey, his parents discuss how severe their son's migraines have become with the other parents. One of the adults asks if they have tried chiropractic. The boy's parents respond, "No, the doctors have never mentioned anything about that." One of the fathers says he is a chiropractor and maybe he can help their son. Although they don't know much about chiropractic, it is too difficult to watch their boy suffer. They are ready to try anything.

The next time their son has a migraine, they call the chiropractor and rush him to the chiropractor's office. The chiropractor does an assessment and performs an adjustment. Almost miraculously, for the first time since the injury, the young boy experiences relief from the headache. After fifteen minutes, the pain is gone and he is playing street hockey with his friends!

This dramatic story is about me and how chiropractic saved my life! My discovery of health through chiropractic inspired me to become a chiropractor and devote the rest of my life to helping others.

**H**ow many people feel confident about placing their health and wellness in the hands of the provincial or stateun healthcare system? Do you think there is no need to vorry? If you get sick, will you rely on the government to take are of you? Does that seem like a good idea?

Wait times in Canada are at an all-time high because of ignificant pressure on our medical manpower and facilities. Ve are in a healthcare crisis because of the current sickness rends in our aging population. As baby boomers enter their ixties and the disease care model continues to demand xtreme financial support, the western world economy will ot be able to keep up with the current level of spending.

How confident are you that you won't die before you get he necessary medical service? Medical wait times are forcng many Canadians to go to private clinics, or even other ountries, to have medical procedures performed sooner.

How confident do you feel placing your health and wellless in the hands of pharmaceutical companies? In our resent system, we know they wield much financial power.

If you are confident in this model of healthcare, I invite ou to take a look at how the pharmaceutical industry is perorming. In 2003, the *Canadian Medical Association Journal* evealed that 38,000 people died due to adverse side effects rom properly prescribed medicines. That means the right rug, for the right condition, at the intended dosage, killed 8,000 people! And the *Journal of the American Medical ssociation* reports an estimated 28 percent of all hospital dmissions are due to problems caused by physiologically ncompatible prescription drugs.

There is increasing awareness of pharmaceutical companies withholding information from research studies on the afety of their drugs. This includes misinforming medical docors who distribute or prescribe them.

A classic example is the drug Vioxx, an anti-inflammatory rug in the non-steroidal anti-inflammatory class, similar to aspirin and ibuprofen. Vioxx was marketed worldwide, pre scribed to more than 20 million people, with 2003 reporte sales of $2.5 billion. Studies revealed that those who ha taken Vioxx had double the risk of suffering a heart attack Despite preliminary studies showing a risk for cardiovascula events, Merck, the pharmaceutical company that produce Vioxx, still heavily marketed the drug. Finally, in Septembe 2004, Merck withdrew Vioxx from the market, making it th largest drug recall in history.

A study published in the prestigious medical journal *Th Lancet,* authored by Dr. Graham, found that 140,000 cases c heart disease in the United States and 58,000 deaths wer caused by Vioxx during its five years on the market. It i seemingly obvious that pharmaceutical companies are mor concerned about their bottom-line profits than the health an well-being of our community.

In 2005, The Center of Public Integrity reported that mos pharmaceutical companies spend more on marketing than o research. Mega-producers Pfizer and GlaxoSmithKlin topped the list by spending twice as much on marketing tha they did on research. Pfizer spent $16.9 billion on marketin and $7.68 billion on research, while GlaxoSmithKline sper $12.93 billion on marketing and $5.20 billion on research Do you trust the pharmaceutical industry with your health?

Most of us were taught to hold medical doctors o pedestals and not to question their recommendations Realizing that much of the information utilized by physician is actually provided by pharmaceutical companies, are yo willing to put your health and wellness in the hands of you medical doctor?

Let's take a look at how medical doctors are performing The *Canadian Medical Association Journal* exposed that 40,00 people die in hospitals due to preventable medical error. Thi statistic only relates to hospitals—it does not include private practices.

The number one killer in Canada is heart disease, which takes approximately 100,000 lives each year. If you combine the 38,000 deaths caused by adverse effects to medications and the 40,000 people who die due to medical errors in hospitals, you discover that 78,000 deaths per year are preventable. And, as I already stated, this number does not account for private practice errors. (Presumably not all preventable deaths are appropriately accounted for. This would just be bad business.) Personally, I would be extremely reluctant to enter our present medical system unless it was an emergency.

The *Journal of the American Medical Association* published that a whopping 250,000 deaths per year are caused by preventable medical errors in hospitals alone. That is the third leading cause of death in the United States, second only to cancer and heart disease!

How many of you feel confident relying on that system?

With the advent of the Internet, consumers have an abundance of health information available to them. In general, the population is more knowledgeable than ever before. Many people go to their doctors' offices with a list of potential diagnoses based on their symptoms and information they've acquired online. What most people seek is a drug or surgery—because they know little else of what is available to them.

The information presented in this chapter is not meant to bash our government or medical doctors, it is solely meant to educate you and open your eyes to the actual picture of the system in which we live. In fact, I am grateful that we have government funding for healthcare, and I sincerely believe that most doctors want to help people and have the best interests of their patients in mind.

However, medical doctors can only perform to the level of their competence based on what they have been taught; and their education is flawed because it focuses on what needs to be added to (medication) or taken away from (surgery) the body to help people be healthy. Note: there is no doubt that medical doctors and hospitals serve a purpose in times of crisis; but true healthcare that improves the quality of life is not what they offer.

The way the human body adapts to lifestyles and chosen behaviors is nothing short of a miracle. People across the western world are under enormous stress. Obesity levels are at an all-time high; smoking, alcohol, and drug consumption is soaring; and more people suffer from insomnia and depression than ever before. Yet, somehow, the human body adapts and maintains its functions, often with dysfunction that is hidden and unapparent—until one day your body starts to breakdown and symptoms appear.

This is when the medical system kicks in, which for many people may be too late. In such instances, we accuse the human body of being "unintelligent," i.e., it has a chemical imbalance or an excess of body parts, and thus major interventions are suggested.

It is wiser to respect the body, understand how intelligent it is, and believe that it always responds to the demands placed upon it. If we chose to discover what causes the body to breakdown, a solution would be imminent and suffering would decrease, putting an end to this healthcare crisis.

Clearly people aren't sick because of a lack of medicine, and they are rarely born with too many body parts. People are sick because they make sick choices. These choices force our bodies to adapt, driving us into a state of dis-ease. If this dis-ease persists for a prolonged period of time, our bodies will breakdown further.

Symptoms do not occur by mistake; they appear to tell you to make changes to your internal environment and to make better choices for your health. Symptoms are not to be suppressed; they are a manifestation of the cause, just like the oil or engine light in your car. When your engine light turns on, should you ignore the light, unplug the fuse, or pay attention to the warning? If you ignore the light, does the problem typically get better or worse? The answer to this one is quite simple, isn't it? You pay attention and get your vehicle checked and repaired, or more serious problems occur.

Disease is the result of a breakdown in adaptation, when the organism can no longer cope with excessive demands from its environment. If changes are not made, sickness leading to death is the ultimate result.

When you visit your medical doctor, what are you looking for? Do you want something to relieve a symptom or something to help you get well? Does high blood pressure medicine help you regain your health so that you can stop taking it? No, you will most likely take it for the rest of your life.

Is this in *your* best interest or that of the pharmaceutical company that manufactures the drug?

What if there were other options? Would you be willing to consider a new model for true health? It should be evident that health doesn't come from a pill, just as money doesn't grow on trees. Do people experience headaches because they have a lack of Tylenol in their system? Sounds foolish to ask such a question, doesn't it?

I had severe headaches, and not until the cause of the symptom was discovered and corrected did I rediscover health. People are not sick because they are born with a lack of drugs in their body, nor are they sick because they were born with too many body parts.

For years, doctors removed tonsils thinking they were causing sore throats. In reality, having swollen tonsils is just a symptom of the cause of the problem. Many of us know people who had their tonsils removed, yet this intervention had no effect on the number of sore throats they experienced. Tonsils serve an important role in immune system function by producing cells—T-lymphocytes—that actually help you get rid of infections. Without tonsils, you lose an important avenue to ward off infection.

You are taught that when you are sick you go to the doctor and he or she cures you. In reality, there is only one thing that can cure you—the innate intelligence within you, a wisdom that, through your nervous system, controls and coordinates the one hundred trillion cells in your body. This innate intelligence is responsible for every physiological function that takes place within you! Even when medical professionals apply an intervention, it is still your innate intelligence that does the healing. What happens when you apply a medical intervention to a corpse? Nothing, of course. Can you think of any more scientific evidence needed to make this point?

Life heals! The inner wisdom inside living beings dictates healing.

The definition of *insanity* is doing the same thing over and over again while expecting a different result. We need to look no further than our senior population to get an illustration of this insanity. Would you say our seniors are the healthiest population you've ever looked at? Of course not! Many people are afraid of living into their sixties and seventies because they see the suffering. Our elderly population has been getting sicker and sicker every year; yet, we continue to do the exact same things when it comes to health. This is insane!

When I speak to groups, one of my favorite questions to

ask is: "How many of you would like to grow up to live like your parents or grandparents?" When they balk at raising their hands, I then ask what they are doing to ensure poor health will not happen to them.

Our seniors grew up in an era when they entrusted their health and well-being to the government and the medical community (which is strongly influenced by the pharmaceutical industry). Most adults took little to no responsibility for their health. When they became sick, they relied on the system to cure them. Yet, they have been getting sicker, suffering more, and draining the so-called healthcare system. I sincerely believe this is not by choice but simply ignorance.

Who can we blame for this lack of education?

The Public Health Agency of Canada reports that the average adult over sixty-five takes up to 4.5 different medications. I have had patients walk into my office with shopping bags of medication; some taking more than eighteen different meds at one time! Many seniors are prescribed medications to alleviate the side effects of other medications.

When researchers study a particular drug, they try to isolate all other variables so they can identify how the drug affects a certain condition. Therefore, they are not studying the interaction of multiple medications on an individual's overall health. According to *Health Canada*, seniors comprise 13 percent of our population and account for 44.4 percent of all deaths due to adverse drug reactions. *Health Canada* also noted that, when compared to the rest of the population, drug use was significantly higher among seniors accounting for 40 percent of all medications consumed.

Continuing on this path of destruction will not only create more suffering, it will bankrupt our economy. We desperately need to change this attitude toward healthcare and start taking responsibility for our own health. If you don't respect yourself enough to start making changes, you are bound for disaster and there is little hope for humanity!

Some seniors have chosen not to follow the norm and have taken responsibility for their health by choosing to exercise, take vitamins, eat healthy, and develop stress-reduction mechanisms. Are these the people in nursing homes? No, these people are enjoying their Golden Years and living vibrant, healthy lives. They contribute to society and spend time with their grandchildren. They are an asset to the world, providing support, wisdom, and hope.

Why don't more people look at these healthy adults as examples for good living and choose to make similar choices? It is time that we educated and empowered people to take responsibility for themselves so that they, too, can create lives of health and well-being rather than lives of sickness and disease.

We are a reactionary society, waiting until we get sick or have symptoms before we act. We determine our health based on how we feel. If we feel good, we must be healthy. However, heart disease and cancer, the top killers in North America, are conditions that progress for years asymptomatically. In other words, the condition is destroying someone's health and they don't even know it.

The most common symptom of heart disease is sudden death. That means no one knew this person had an illness until he or she suddenly had a heart attack and died!

One day you FEEL perfectly healthy on the golf course, the next day you are dead from a heart attack. Is that the kind of life you want or deserve? People can have grapefruit-size tumors in their intestines before they FEEL any symptoms. How you feel and look is a poor barometer of how healthy you are. Skinny people have heart attacks, too.

We can no longer wait until crisis occurs before we react.

We must be proactive and do whatever it takes to stay out of our current sick-care system, while at the same time be grateful that the system exists in case of a crisis.

Taking pills is passive and easy—true healthcare takes effort. Our medical model serves to treat disease. It does not promote wellness. Passive healthcare has not worked and will never be effective at maintaining your health and preventing disease, even though it may save your life in an emergency.

What will you do to stay out of the current sick-care system?

Ultimately, health is a simple concept. What would you tell obese people to do to get well? Modify their diet, exercise daily, reduce stress, and ensure their nervous system is functioning optimally are wise suggestions. These recommendations are no different for someone with heart disease, cancer, or diabetes. Those conditions are also a manifestation of the same cause . . . poor lifestyle choices!

You have been led to believe that most conditions are the result of your genes; and there is nothing you can do about your genetics. Realize, most diseases are degenerative in nature, meaning the breakdown occurs slowly, over many years. These conditions—most cancers, heart disease, and type II diabetes—have little to do with your genetic makeup. They are the adaptation of your body to poor lifestyle choices for so long that your body begins to break down.

Even though multiple members of a family suffer from similar conditions, it is not because of bad genes. It is because they are brought up in similar environments and make similar lifestyle choices. If disease was based on genetics, then everyone in a family would have the condition, wouldn't they?

The whole gene concept has been studied extensively.

When identical twins are brought up in completely different environments, they have different disease presentations. Their environments and lifestyles are better indicators of what types of illness may manifest, especially regarding cancer, heart disease, and diabetes—the most common diseases of adaptation.

We can no longer take the easy road and blame our genes; this theory has little substance. Human genes haven't changed much in the last 40,000 years, but our lifestyle has. Our genes have stayed the same, yet the expression of these genes has changed drastically due to the environments we expose ourselves to.

In many ways, the general population is under more stress than ever. And people don't eat as healthy or exercise as often as they should. Genes cannot be blamed for how your body adapts to your lifestyle. Your body adapts to the environment it is exposed to and the response your body has to its environment is incredibly intelligent. If you go for a run, what happens to your blood pressure? It goes up. Is that an error? Are you sick? Should you take a pill? No, that is the body's response to the metabolic demands of the environment. The innate intelligence within you ALWAYS adapts appropriately to the environment.

Your goal should be to respect that response and to provide your body with the best potential to heal, with the ultimate goal of adding as much health to the system as possible, so your body has the highest probability to function optimally. You face many environmental stressors that are unavoidable; however, the healthier your body is, the better able you are to adapt to these stressors.

Improve the environment within you and you will be better suited to adapt to the environment around you. Treat your body like a temple and it will show you miracles.

Do you ever wonder why certain people frequently get sick, while others don't? Why does one person in your family come down with the flu but no one else does? If you are exposed to their germs, wouldn't you catch it, too?

Most people have microbes within them; the issue is whether your immune system can control the microbes so you don't manifest symptoms. If your system is overwhelmed with internal stress, the energy it has for healing, growth, and repair is limited. Cancer, for example, is mostly an immune issue. All of us have cancer cells in us right now. What prevents you from experiencing the disease is how effectively your immune system can prevent the cancer cells from reproducing and multiplying.

If you want to be healthy, you have to provide yourself with what is genetically required for you to be healthy. The fundamental question is: What are the genetic requirements for a human being to express health? If every cell in your body functions optimally, you would rarely get sick. If sickness manifests, something must be interfering with your body's natural ability to express health.

When your dog is sick, you probably wonder what it ate. Did it wander out of the yard and get into something unusual? Yet, when you are sick, the most common question is: Did you take anything for it?

Shouldn't you be looking for what may have caused the illness instead of searching for what you can do to eliminate the symptom? What did you do that inhibited your body's natural healing ability? What did you eat last week? Have you been exercising regularly or have you lived a sedentary lifestyle? Are you practicing proper stress-relieving techniques?

Most people look for external solutions that have nothing to do with the cause of the problem, they only seek to mask the symptom. The requirements for a healthy body are simple: a healthy diet, physical exercise, controlled stress, and a properly functioning nervous system.

What is a healthy diet? You could refer to the Canadian Food Guide as a resource; however, it is not based on research. The Canadian Food Guide is heavily influenced by lobby groups, with the base of the pyramid recommending that most of your daily consumption should be from grains and dairy products.

According to research, though, a diet high in grains and dairy is significantly related to increased incidences of heart disease, cancer, Type II diabetes, and even osteoporosis. Unfortunately, the dairy and grain farmers have heavily influenced our political policymakers.

Research reveals that people with low incidences of heart disease, diabetes, cancer, osteoporosis, and many of the common ailments of today, have diets that consist of vegetables and fruit, some nuts, protein mostly from chicken and fish, and some red meat. Very little grain and essentially no dairy products outside of the mother's breast milk is consumed.

Humans are the only mammals that drink milk from another mammal, and I don't know of any other mammals with osteoporosis. The majority of your diet should come from vegetables and each meal should contain some protein. If you want to be healthy, start each day with a breakfast primarily made up of fruit and vegetables with some protein. A blended shake is a great way to combine these ingredients!

Before lunch and dinner add a salad with a variety of raw and cooked veggies accompanied by an animal source of protein. Try to eat frequently, six to eight small meals per day; with lots of water, approximately four litres, in between.

These simple modifications will provide your body with

the nutrients it needs to express wellness. I also recommend supplementation for nutrients that you cannot get from your diet. For example, the North American diet is almost completely devoid of omega 3 fatty acids. Therefore, it is important that you supplement with high quality fish oil. Innate Choice is an incredible product by Dr. James Chestnut, one of my mentors. His research is the root of much of the information I have shared in this section.

It is wise to take a high quality multivitamin because soils where fruits and vegetables are grown have become devoid of many of the essential nutrients required for health. If fruits and vegetables contained the nutrients they once did, you wouldn't need to supplement because you would get all the vitamins from your diet in a whole food source, which is best. A multivitamin is just a top up. Remember, you eat healthy not to look good or to lose weight but to give your body the best opportunity to function.

It is incredibly important to exercise daily. This doesn't mean you have to run a marathon, but you need to do some form of activity every day. Many little things, like taking the stairs instead of the elevator, parking farther away and walking, add up. Try to do a variety of exercise, from flexibility or yoga, strength training, Pilates, and cardiovascular or aerobic. The body benefits from all types activity. To express health you require regular exercise.

Stress has a huge impact on your health; therefore, finding appropriate ways to reduce stress will have tremendous benefits. There are many techniques available; it is important that you discover what works best for you. Exercise is probably one of the best ways to control stress. Other suggestions include meditation, visualization, reading, goal setting, time management, planning, making lists, purposeful living, and letting go of fears and guilt.

Be grateful for what you have. Being grateful attracts more of what you are grateful for.

Be humble. The definition of *humble* that I like is "the degree to which you see yourself in others." Start by loving yourself first and look for characteristics of yourself in others. If someone cuts you off while you are driving, ask yourself if you ever cut someone off, even by error. Of course, nobody is perfect. Love people for who they are and for their unique differences. Remember the law of attraction states that whatever you focus on you attract into your life. Try not dwell on problems, and instead choose to focus on solutions.

In chiropractic, we understand the fact that your body is a self-healing, self-regulating organism and your nervous system is the master system that controls and coordinates the vital life force. Chiropractors recognize that interference in your nervous system decreases your body's ability to function optimally. We know that nerve interference creates more stress within you and your nervous system has to attend to it, disrupting the health, growth, and repair functions. These stressful impulses take precedence as your nervous system places them higher on the survival hierarchy.

For example, if you are stranded outside in a snowstorm your body will pool blood away from the extremities to your core to ensure that the vital organs get the necessary blood supply to keep you alive; the hierarchy being that in an emergency like this you need your vital organs more than your foot.

Your body is so intelligent it will virtually sacrifice its own tissue for the survival of the whole. In understanding this hierarchy and intelligence, chiropractors do not focus on changing the internal environment of the body but rather ensuring its proper functioning. Again, if every cell in your body was functioning optimally, you would not get sick.

Therefore, to remove the interfered and distorted nerve impulses, chiropractors look to the spine since it is the most highly nerve-dense area in the body. Every adjustment performed by a chiropractor sends a healthy impulse to the brain called *proprioception*. These proprioceptive (good) inputs override the stressful or nociceptive (not so good) inputs from fixated or misaligned spinal joints, thus creating healthier outputs.

As your brain receives more healthy input, it produces more healthy growth and repair output. The old adage of garbage in, garbage out, or good in, good out, definitely relates to nervous system output and ultimate health results.

As a result of chiropractic adjustments and normalized nervous system function, many patients have experienced miraculous global health changes, not because chiropractic is a specific treatment or cure for these conditions, but because chiropractic adjustments increase your health potential and allow your body a greater opportunity to heal. If you eat bad sushi and you begin to vomit, is this an unhealthy response? Should you try to suppress the vomiting? No, this is a healthy response! If you don't get rid of the toxicity, it could kill you! Many people choose to take something when they don't feel well and this interferes with the body's natural healing abilities.

Did you know that many microbes cannot reproduce in a temperature between 102 and 104 degrees Fahrenheit and, since they have a life span of twenty-four to forty-eight hours, when the body temperature is elevated for this time period the microbes that are noxious to your body die; and since they were unable to reproduce your body becomes well? Should you take an aspirin to reduce your fever if that is the natural response of the body?

Chiropractic is the foundation of health, as all other components are completely dependent upon the proper functioning of the nervous system. When your nervous system is at optimal function, you will experience the true benefits of a healthy diet, exercise, and reduced stress.

Believe in yourself and take action today to create the healthiest body you can. Don't focus on the past, look to improve the future. Take responsibility for your health today and healing will begin tomorrow! Respect your inner wisdom and it will show you miracles.

You can contact Dr. D. J. LeDrew at:

Full Potential Chiropractic
#11, 5308 17th Ave SW
Calgary, Alberta, Canada T3E 6S6
Phone: 403-204-0084
Email: fullpotential@shaw.ca

www.fullpotentialchiro.com

8.

# Unexplained Fatigue

## James D. Powell, DC

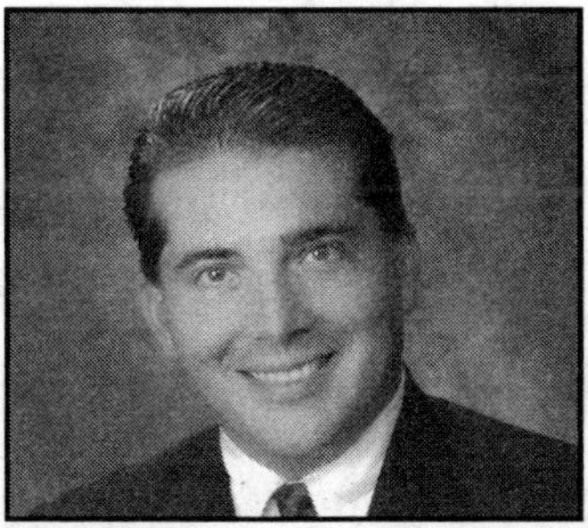

I am a second generation chiropractor. My family first became aware of the value of chiropractic when my dad's mother became paralyzed after being inoculated with a mandatory polio vaccine in the early 1950s. Fortunately, my grandmother was a determined Scottish woman and was committed to walking again. She sought out many different types of practitioners, speaking to anyone who might be able to help her achieve her goal of walking again. As God would have it, she stumbled upon a chiropractor who accepted her as a patient.

This chiropractor's office was on the second floor, so every day my grandfather and father carried my grandmother up two flights of stairs and into the treatment room. Once my grandmother had received her adjustment, they would carry her back down, repeating this with love and dedication three times a week for months.

After about nine weeks of regular care, my grandmother excitedly told her chiropractor that she was regaining feeling and mobility in her toes. She eventually recovered completely, as some would say "against all odds." It was absolutely amazing. Upon hearing her story I was deeply touched and always wondered how this chiropractor performed such a feat.

Now, to my story. My father and mother married when they were both twenty-one. Immediately after the wedding, they moved to Lombard, Illinois, so that my father could pursue a degree in chiropractic. Shortly thereafter, they learned my mother was pregnant. My parents were excited about the birth of their first child.

When my dad learned my mother was in labor, he drove to the hospital as fast as he could. He anticipated being witness to a simple, miraculous event.

However, during labor, my mother developed severe cramping in her abdomen and lower back, which refused to pass no matter what was tried. With the encouragement of a well-meaning nurse practitioner and obstetrician, Mom agreed to an epidural injection.

For an epidural to be fully effective it must be given at the appropriate time and the dose must be calculated to last until the child is born. Unfortunately, my mother's ability to process the medication was faster than the doctor had calculated. The epidural wore off too soon. Mom labored for twenty-four hours and received three separate epidurals during this time period. (This was not standard practice in the 1960s nor is it standard medical practice today.)

My father and mother were horrified by the sight of their first child—a completely dark-blue baby. What a sight to behold! They knew their son was either in crisis, or maybe dead. The infant had been exposed to too many epidural injections, which caused decreased blood flow and oxygen content to his body, to the point where he turned blue. (Usually when a baby is born blue, it is dead.) The baby was revived, of course; otherwise I wouldn't be telling my story. Yes, the baby I am talking about is me.

I am told that I did not utter a sound when I was born, not a cry or a whimper. After spending some time underneath an oxygen tent, I went home. Even though my parents took good care of me, by my first birthday it was evident that something was significantly wrong. I was lethargic, small, and not active like most children my age.

At my first birthday party, well-meaning friends and family allowed me to consume the majority of an iced cake. The sugar overload caused an almost immediate asthmatic attack in me, and once again my parents were subject to the frightening sight of a blue baby. Fortunately, we were within five blocks of the local hospital.

I am told my father picked me up and actually ran to the hospital with me in his arms. In the ER department, I was taken from my parents. After a long, torturous wait, the ER physician presented in the waiting room where Mom and Dad had stood for what seemed to them to be eternity. My parents were told that they had almost lost their son and that significant precautions would have to be in place to prevent such future events from occurring. There was concern of allergies and the effects that severe allergic reactions can create on the respiratory system, sending a child into respiratory distress and often causing death.

My parents had to keep me away from strong perfumes and other potent odors, especially cigarette smoke. Imagine the challenge. This was the 1960s and early 1970s, when the majority of people smoked.

It became difficult for my parents to protect me from all these environmental pollutants. Where could they take me to keep me safe? They were both fearful of exposing me to any situation that could cause me to suffer another life-threatening asthmatic attack. During the first few months after that initial hospital visit, my asthma attacks became more frequent and visits to the emergency room became the norm.

The ER physicians and the pediatrician that examined me prepared my parents for the reality that I was unlikely to live beyond nine years old and would certainly not live a normal life or be able to participate in any athletic sport. My parents were directed to shelter me from the outside world.

My parents had no health insurance, so the mounting bills, stress, and the fear of finding me dead in my crib became overwhelming. My father, who was attending chiropractic college fulltime and working a part-time job, started to fall asleep during his classes. Thankfully, one day his teacher kindly asked, "Is there something that I could be of assistance with? What seems to be the problem?"

When my father explained the situation, this teacher boldly and courageously suggested that my father not take me to the hospital during my next attack. Instead, he offered to care for me himself.

Now, let's consider for a moment the importance of his offer. This teacher took a stand on the issue of my asthma by daring to suggest that my parents not take me to the emergency department the next time I had an attack. He knew with certainty that chiropractic could help me and that there was something he would be able to do. However, by making this offer, he risked his license and his job as a chiropractic college teacher.

A few days later, I suffered another asthmatic attack. My mother and father jumped in the car and raced to this doctor of chiropractic's house. Imagine how fearful my parents must have been. They had never experienced the true magnificence of chiropractic as it relates to children and they must have wondered if going there was a mistake, considering that their child was in respiratory distress.

My parents had no idea what kind of treatment I would receive. All they knew was that I was blue and this man said he could help.

The doctor's hands were so large and thick that he provided a significant chiropractic thrust. My father and mother recall that the noises that emanated from my spine while I was adjusted were sounds that they had never heard before, and it frightened them. My mom screamed.

Immediately after the specific chiropractic adjustment to my mid-dorsal spine, I vomited the most putrid, disgusting fluid that anybody had ever seen. Inside this fluid were small, round, shell-like structures that today my father recognizes as Kushman's Spirals. Kushman's Spirals are masses of matter that are found in the fluids that asthmatics cough up.

This event lead to the discovery that I had been so drugged at birth from the epidurals my mother received, that I had been unable to develop a cough reflex. As a result, embryonic fluid entered my lungs and remained there for more than eighteen months. Yes, my lungs were sick.

My first chiropractic adjustment stimulated my nervous system to release this foreign matter from my lungs and allowed me to take my first true breath of life. My parents said that after I finished vomiting, I took the deepest breath they had ever seen or heard. And, my body quickly changed color to the normal pink that is seen in other children. They had never seen me look healthy before!

In that moment, my parents knew they had made the right decision to trust this doctor of chiropractic and the human body's innate ability to heal itself. That first chiropractic adjustment changed our lives and rescued me from the dismal future that had been predicted.

My father continued his studies with more focus and determination than ever. He had seen me become healthy and was committed to making a difference in the world. He graduated from chiropractic college and began his practice in Canton, Ohio, in 1971. He was passionate to help children suffering from asthma. The first twenty-five asthmatic children he assessed and adjusted completely recovered. He knew that chiropractic worked in helping sick people get well.

As chiropractic relates to me, I have not experienced another asthmatic attack since that day. The evidence of the power of chiropractic is me being able to write this book and having my picture forefront and center, showing that I am well. I would not be alive had it not been for chiropractic.

Without reservation I say that chiropractic is not only a profession, it is a lifestyle. And in this lifestyle, God has blessed us to participate in and experience miracles. This is why I have chosen to be a chiropractor and a chiropractic patient for life.

Although life can be complicated; there is one simple truth: the human body has the ability to heal itself provided there is no interference. When you cut your finger it is neither the Band-Aid nor the antibiotic cream that repairs the tissue; it is the power of the body.

Chiropractic is a tool that helps the body heal itself. Doctors don't heal; they are simply instruments that facilitate change and healing. Healing doesn't come from the medicine or the herb or the pill or the lotion. It comes from within.

In the textbook *Gray's Anatomy*, which is an important tool for most, if not all, medical and chiropractic college students, it states that the nervous system is the master system that controls all other systems of the body. After basic sciences have been properly learned and tested, however, the separation between medicine and chiropractic becomes clear. Medicine is symptom-based and focuses on the use of medication or surgery to alleviate symptoms. Chiropractic takes a different approach.

After learning the functions of the human body, chiropractic doctors are taught spinal adjusting, physical therapy modulation, nutrition, and other forms of natural interventions to assist the body in healing and maintaining health. These are separate and distinct types of health-care interventions—even though the fundamentals are the same.

When chiropractors look at the nervous system, we first consider how the brain and spinal cord are functioning and communicating with the rest of the body. The brain and spinal cord make up the central nervous system and all nerve structures outside the skull and spine are referred to as the *peripheral nervous system*. The brain is a living tissue that produces a certain amount of electrical current and this electrical current passes out of the skull, down through your spinal column, into the brain stem and spinal cord and is distributed throughout the body via the peripheral nervous system.

The spinal column is made up of twenty-four moveable bones with twenty-four separate pairs of nerve roots. These nerves are important "communication cables" between your body and your brain.

I have used the following analogy with many patients over the years: If you connect your computer to a printer, the computer would be the brain and the printer would be an end unit/organ that is receiving information via a cable, which in your body is a nerve. In your body, your brain communicates with your adrenal and all other glands, muscles, and organs. Everything is directly or indirectly linked to the brain. Each organ or tissue receiving information is an end unit. The printer cannot print a document on its own without receiving information from the computer. The same principle applies to any organ, muscle, or tissue and your brain.

In reviewing the diagram, you will see that the cervical spine (neck) is made up of seven vertebrae (neck bones) and is bent forward 18°. The mid-back or thoracic spine has bones and is bent 36° towards the back. The lumbar spine or lower back has five bones and also has an 18° curve toward the stomach.

When you look at the spine from the side, it resembles a slight S. Physicists have discovered that the body's ability to maintain its weight in gravity and to handle significant compression force is related to this S-curve.

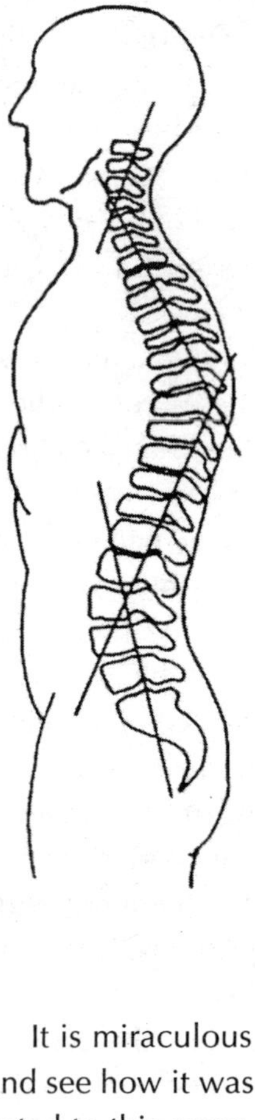

In other words, this curve distributes the body's weight evenly through all the bones of the spine and is able to withstand approximately one hundred times the force that it could if it was straight. Thus, whenever this curve is absent, you are at significant risk. (A straight spine from the back, however, is good.)

Let's look briefly again at the numbers. The neck has seven bones and the lower back has five bones; both bent forward. Seven plus five equals twelve and there are twelve bones bent in the other direction. The neck and the back both curve forward 18°, the mid-back curves backward 36°. Eighteen plus eighteen equals thirty-six, which is 36° going the other direction, so the spine offsets itself.

It is miraculous to look at the structure of your own body and see how it was created. The physics of it cannot be duplicated to this same degree.

The brain communicates with the body through various sets of cables, the cables being spinal nerves. Each nerve has a specific area of the body that it communicates with; so, in utilizing the computer/printer analogy, if the printer cable from the computer isn't plugged in completely the printer will malfunction. If, for example, one of the nerve roots coming out of your back that goes to your adrenal gland has been disrupted, your adrenal gland is likely to malfunction. Decreased power, decreased function.

A relatively easy concept to follow, isn't it?

A chiropractic doctor identifies imbalance in the spine, looks for irritations to the nervous system, and determines how to best correct these issues. Upon relief of the irritation, the body's communication is restored.

Let's go back to when I was eighteen months old and suffering from regular asthma attacks with embryonic fluid in my lungs. The wise chiropractor adjusts my spine and restores proper communication between my lungs and my brain. As soon as my brain identifies the location of the unwanted fluid and matter, it is expelled. Would that have happened if I were using an inhaler or other asthma medication?

No. My body's ability to communicate with itself was disrupted. The chiropractor unlocked the joints of my spine, thereby releasing the nerve root to function and communicate properly.

A chiropractic adjustment saved my life. A chiropractic adjustment could save your life or that of a loved one. It is my sincere desire that the knowledge you gain by reading this book will give you a clear understanding of the importance of proper spinal health.

When a spinal joint is out of its normal position, this phenomenon is called a *subluxation*. Let's examine the meaning of this word. *Sub* is a prefix that means "just beneath or less than." *Ation* is a suffix that means "condition of," and *lux* means "energy or light." Thus, subluxation means "a condition of less light or less energy." Subluxations interfere with the transmission of energy, therefore they affect function.

Please refer to the safety pin diagram on the adjacent page to visualize how the body's communication system is simple to understand. At the top of the safety pin are brain cells and at the bottom are tissue cells. The *afferent pathway* (a pathway of information going *to* the brain) and *efferent pathway* (going *from* the brain) are the edges of the safety pin. These show that a brain cell receives information from a tissue cell or system that something needs to be done, and then the brain sends information down the efferent side to tell the tissue cell what to do. If the safety pin is opened up and the brain cannot communicate accurately with the tissue cell, dysfunction occurs and, in time, a disease process takes place.

In simple terms, subluxation is a safety pin that is open. The chiropractic doctor performs a spinal adjustment to reposition the vertebra and reclose the safety pin. Once fixed, the required power is back on and communication between the brain and the tissue cells is reestablished.

This is the basis for chiropractic; a principle that has stood the test of time. As Pastor John Hampton from Canton, Ohio said: "Practices are many, principles are few. Principles never change, practices always do."

It is imperative that the human race discover the true principle of chiropractic and embark on a quest to great health and wellness.

In our office, we use the phrase "sick and tired of being sick and tired" to describe one of the most common, yet most misdiagnosed, conditions that afflict people worldwide. We believe that the majority of unexplained fatigued patients have a syndrome called *adrenal fatigue*. Although many physi-

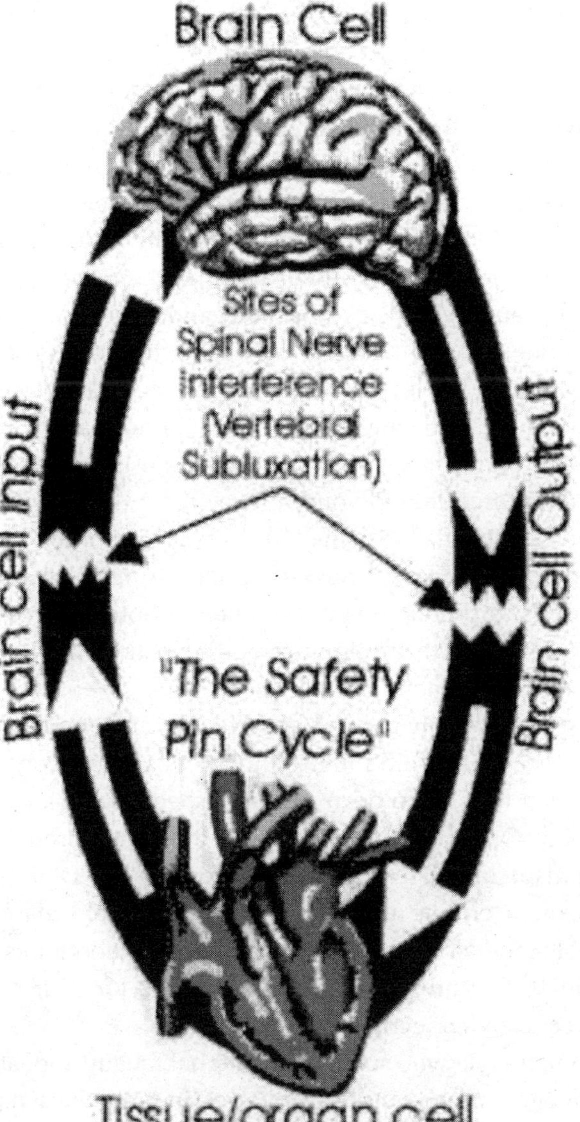
Brain Cell
Sites of
Spinal Nerve
interference
(Vertebral
Subluxation)
Brain cell input
Brain cell Output
"The Safety
Pin Cycle"
Tissue/organ cell

cians throughout the century have utilized terms such as *adrenal fatigue* to describe this affliction, it has not attracted the attention of conventional medicine. Yet it is a significant problem that begs to be addressed.

*Adrenal fatigue* has been defined as "a collection of signs and symptoms that result from the adrenal gland operating below necessary levels." A simple acute infection or a long-standing infection can cause this syndrome, as well as trauma, malnourishment, stress—and the most important cause, in my opinion, is subluxations of the spine.

If you are feeling sick and tired and your symptoms are due to unexplained fatigue, you might choose to rest more, reduce your stress levels, start to eat correctly, exercise more often, or take medication; but, if you do not have your subluxations corrected via chiropractic adjustments, you will never find resolution to your fatigue.

The adrenal gland is small and sits on top of the kidneys. It is no bigger than a walnut and weighs as much as grape. Its purpose is to produce multiple different hormones and hormone precursors that help your body function. One of these hormones is adrenaline.

You are probably familiar with the story of a mother lifting a car to save her child's life. Although this sounds unreasonable, such feats have been accomplished due to adrenaline overload. Other hormones secreted from the adrenal gland are cortisol and DHEA. Measuring cortisol and DHEA levels in saliva determine the health of your adrenal gland. The adrenal gland also produces three precursor hormones, starting blocks that are required in your blood for your body to produce or utilize certain other chemicals.

Some people who suffer from adrenal fatigue appear to be very healthy on the outside. However, in time, the symptoms can be devastating. How can you tell if you are suffering from adrenal fatigue? In his book *Adrenal Fatigue*, Dr. James Wilson lists six symptoms you should look for:

- Tired for no reason
- Trouble getting up in the morning, even when you go to bed at a reasonable hour
- Feeling run-down or overwhelmed
- Can't bounce back from stress or illness
- Crave salty or sweet snacks
- Feeling best after 6:00 P.M.

Adrenal fatigue is close to my heart because I experienced it firsthand. Early in my chiropractic career, it took every ounce of my energy to go from one treatment room to the next. I had symptoms I did not understand and there appeared to be no reason for these issues. I was young, looked fit, slept a lot; yet I found it harder and harder to get out of bed.

I would search out coffee or sugar to give me a stimulant between 9:30 a.m. and 11:00 a.m. and between 3:00 p.m. and 5:00 p.m. If I stayed up past 11:30 p.m., I would then experience a second wind and could virtually stay up all night.

I went to school thirty-four hours per week, spent multiple hours studying, and worked full-time as a waiter to help pay for my education. Upon graduation, I immediately went to work in my father's chiropractic clinic. In an attempt to show my gratitude and dedication, I worked fifty-hour weeks and still found time to meet up with my friends at night. Of course, my sleep suffered.

But, I was young, fit, active, and I received regular chiropractic care. I had managed on little sleep while in college, so I thought I still could.

However, because I neglected my sleep and wasn't eating properly, adrenal fatigue syndrome almost overtook me. Fortunately, by utilizing a variety of different resources, which are included in the list of references, I was able to successfully accomplish a proper functioning adrenal gland—but it was not without effort.

What seemed to offer me the greatest benefit were specific chiropractic adjustments of the T9 vertebra. The thoracic vertebra #9 gives rise to the T9 nerve and the T9 nerve goes to the adrenal glands. By receiving a chiropractic adjustment at that level, my adrenal gland benefited from the greatest amount of energy coming from my brain.

My body also needed extra nutritional support to allow me to function at my optimum, so I chose to augment my diet with herbs, vitamins, and a variety of nutritional supplements. My brand of choice is Standard Process, which is only available in a health-care practitioner's office. You should only use nutritional products under the supervision of a health-care advisor.

Another key to recovery is proper rest. This may sound strange, but sleeping in once in awhile is not being lazy. And it is important that you get to sleep before 10:30 p.m. on a regular basis. My wife thought I was crazy trying to go to bed by 9:00 p.m. I didn't do it very often; but when I did, I noticed significant improvement in my level of energy the next day.

Extra sleep will significantly help you recover from many ailments, and it certainly is important if you suffer from unexplained fatigue.

Exercise is another factor in recovering from adrenal fatigue. I know, the most common reason people state for not exercising is fatigue. But, exercise actually helps the body recover and gives you energy.

Different people require different forms of exercise to truly gain the maximum benefit of working out. Some people thrive on high-intensity, high-cardio-aerobic exercise. They probably embrace long-distance running or high-force exertion. Experiencing an elevated heart rate and increasing their metabolism gives them a certain level of relief. They enjoy it. Their bodies operate well at that stage and so they continue doing it.

However, a percentage of the population does not enjoy such intense workouts and, therefore, they need a different style of exercise. Body types vary and each body type requires a separate style of exercise. A chiropractic doctor can help you find the right exercise program for your body type.

We recognize that for many people, the hardest step they have to take is to actually begin exercising. Once a rhythm is established and exercise becomes a habit, it becomes easier.

A wise man once stated: "All of us are victims of our habits." So, replace your bad habits with good ones. Good health habits are worth it. They will add years to your life and life to your years.

In our office, we identify every clients' blood type because this information guides our recommendations for their diet and exercise. For example, Type-O individuals should perform intense physical exercises, like aerobics, martial arts, contact sports, and running. (Type-O happens to be the most common blood type.) Exercise for Type-A individuals should be calming and centering, like yoga and tai chi. Type-B individuals should select moderate physical exercise with mental balance, such as hiking, cycling, tennis, and swimming. Type-AB individuals do well combining calming, centering exercises (yoga and tai chi) with moderate physical exercises (hiking, cycling, and tennis).

There are also certain foods that go with specific blood types. Foods to avoid if you are Type O are wheat, corn, kidney beans, navy beans, lentils, cabbage, brussel sprouts, cauliflower, and mustard greens. Food items that help Type-O individuals with weight loss and balancing the body's nutrition are kelp, seafood, salt, liver, red meat, kale, spinach, and broccoli.

Type-A people should avoid meat, dairy, kidney beans, lima beans, and wheat. Foods that benefit Type-A individuals are vegetable oil, olive oil, soy foods (organic only), vegetables, and pineapple. It is suggested that Type-B people avoid corn, lentils, peanuts, sesame seeds, buckwheat, and wheat; and that they consume greens, eggs, venison, liver, licorice, and tea. Type-AB people should avoid meat, dairy, kidney beans, lima beans, and wheat; and consume vegetable oil, olive oil, soy foods (organic), vegetables, and pineapple.

I hope this information has stimulated you to want to take better care of your most important asset—your health. This book is not meant as a method to diagnose or treat a condition; it is meant to inform you that you may have problems that can be helped by chiropractic adjustments. I encourage you to learn more about your health and to search for answers.

At Powell Chiropractic, we have found that every person who has a spinal misalignment is in desperate need of spinal rehab, especially if they ever hope to recover from a wide variety of ailments. We use a very specific program designed to address the concerns of each individual.

Please know that the team at Powell Chiropractic is here to serve you. Give us a call so we can help you on your road to discovering wellness.

Dr. James Powell
Powell Chiropractic
4867 Munson St. N.W.
Canton, OH 44718
330-494-5533
DrJim@powellchiropractic.com
www.powellchiropractic.com,

## References

D'Adamo. Peter J., *Eat Right for Your Type*, www.dadamo.com

Gray, Henry, *Gray's Anatomy*

Guyton, Dr. Clifton, *Guyton's Physiology*

Wilson, Dr.James, *Adrenal Fatigue: The 21st Century Stress Syndrome*, Smart Publication, 2001

www.StandardProcess.com

www.adrenalfatigue.org

# 9.

# Obtaining Balance In Your Life

## Dr. Nima Rahmany

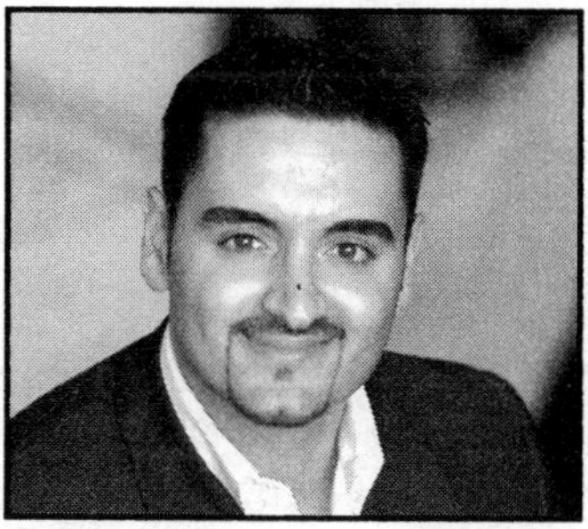

While in the process of establishing a thriving chiropractic practice in less than five years, **Dr. Nima Rahmany** researched universal principles and applied them to his healing techniques and daily living, which resulted in a rapid development in the seven areas of life: spiritual, mental, vocational, financial, social, familial, and physical.

As a student of Dr. John Demartini, a leader in the field of personal transformation and a guest expert on the documentary *The Secret*, Dr. Nima learned how to apply the law of attraction in his chiropractic practice and currently is owner of a multi-disciplinary, complementary health and wellness center. While consulting with his patients on an individual level for stress management, the inevitable shift took place and Dr. Nima became a professional speaker. He created his "Life Skills for a Stressful World" workshop to help people shift their own perceptions from stress to success.

Now, after becoming a stage actor and professional salsa dancer, Dr. Nima continues to expand his personal mission and has already reached thousands of people with his message. He continues to maintain a thriving wellness-based chiropractic practice for families in Maple Ridge, British Columbia.

From a young age, I was aware there were basically two types of people. The first type seemed to be in a chronic depressed mental state, constantly suffering and complaining of aches and pains, sick all the time, functioning with a glass-is-half-empty attitude, and living in a state of turmoil and conflict. Even at five years old, I remember not feeling comfortable around such people and making a conscious choice to live my life differently.

Then, there were people who were happy, healthy, saw life with a glass-is-half-full attitude, spread positivism to those around them, were the life of the party, and were always having fun and living life to its fullest.

I decided to model this latter group because I could see myself as a product of this paradigm of living. Little did I know at the time, however, that his perception of these two polarities would eventually cause me a great deal of stress and inner turmoil.

For many years, the main conflict in my life was caused by questions I asked myself: "Why am I doing so much to be a good person, to be positive, and to help others, while I continually run into chaos, confusion, conflict with friends and family, and depressed states of being? How can I be a good person inside and be so misunderstood at work, with family, friends, and in my relationships?"

My quest for answers led me on a path of self-discovery, self-reflection, and years of post-secondary education. What you are about to read in this chapter are my reflections based on my personal and professional experiences, years of research and learning, and an open heart to truly serve humanity.

> "Living a fulfilling life requires first a definition of what that means for you, taking care of your material and spiritual health before it deteriorates, and transforming your disempowering stressful states into being grateful for whatever is thrown your way."
>
> Dr. Nima Rahmany

As a practicing chiropractor since 2001, I help hundreds of people each and every week. They arrive with low-back pain, neck pain, headaches, numbness and tingling in their extremities, digestive problems, and a multitude of other muscular and skeletal issues. You name it, if it has to do with the human body, I have seen it and dealt with it. (I have even treated a few furry friends! Sometimes people bring in their dog and ask, "Dr. Nima, can you look at Sparky for me?")

Some clients put me on a pedestal; others resent me. I've been judged and labeled, honored and invited as a guest speaker, referred to and quoted, and have had the opportunity to inspire countless people to live healthier lives and to discover their life purpose. As a result of amazing career ups and downs, I have learned much about life, myself, and the human race in general. Seeing my patients experience their stresses, living lessons learned from my various coaches and social contacts, I have discovered valuable pearls of wisdom. I often tell people that if they want to learn about life, about themselves, and about other people, they should become a chiropractor.

I have learned the secret to creating my life exactly the way I want it to be and how to awaken my "inner doctor" to enable my body to heal itself. I now know how much emotions play a role in the overall health of an individual. These discoveries have provided me with the tools necessary to take any stressful situation from the past, present, or future and turn it into a grateful state of empowerment, dissolving inner and outer conflicts as they arise.

My goal is to share these pearls with you.

Because I wanted to be a positive-thinking person and was on a mission to live happily ever after, I took a keen interest in studying the works of great achievers. I became a dedicated fan of Tony Robbins, preaching his words to family and friends. During my university years, I joined a fraternity. As part of this fellowship group, we were forced to read books and provide verbal reports to the rest of the organization, a requirement that some of my fraternity brothers didn't exactly look forward to. As a joke they did talks on "The idiots guide to dating" or "Brewing your own beer;" while I spoke on "Awakening the Giant Within."

My quest for successful living has been helpful in my

practice—the idea that living an extraordinary life is a process that can be mastered with the right amount of examination and deliberate, prioritized action steps. It has even helped me understand my patients.

Many of the issues that patients consult my advice and services for are often the result of inadvertently covering up underlying emotional conflicts. More and more, I am discovering that muscle and joint-related issues can encourage and inspire people to unleash their fears and conflicts, honor themselves (for a change, sometimes), and go out and start living their most inspired lives.

Seldom do I see someone who is constantly sick and tired who doesn't have layers of emotional turmoil as the root cause. Anyone who isn't living his or her purpose is dying—and if you are manifesting a decrease in your health and vitality, it is wise to start listening to what your body is attempting to tell you, so you can begin your journey to healing.

The path towards healing is, in fact, an opportunity for self-discovery.

## Choosing the Right Practitioner

If you are sick and/or in pain, who should you turn to for help? How do you choose the right health-care professional? With so many differing opinions, which one is right for you?

At chiropractic college, I learned how the human body manifests disease and, out of the hundreds of treatment choices available, I learned specific modalities pertaining to adjusting spinal vertebra that are stuck, fixated, out of alignment, or simply do not function as they should. These dysfunctions irritate the nerve roots and cause further dysfunction to more distant tissues and organs. These misaligned vertebras are also known as *subluxations*.

Although all chiropractic doctors have the intention of facilitating the healing process with their patients, there is a division among chiropractors regarding their role in healing. "Mechanistic" doctors of chiropractic believe their role is to set into motion certain "stuck or irritated" spinal segments, thereby promoting greater range of motion in the spine and a decrease in pain. Conversely, the "Vitalistic" doctors of chiropractic believe there is an innate intelligence that is housed within the nervous system. This innate intelligence is transferred from the brain, down the spinal cord, and to all tissues and cells via spinal nerves, and flows from "above-down, inside-out." This innate intelligence is life, and gives life to the body. Interferences to the normal flow of nerve energy, subluxations, disrupt the innate intelligence and lead to dysfunction and, in time, dis-ease, which leads to disease.

The word *subluxation* in medical context refers to a "subtle, partial dislocation." Holistically, *subluxation* can be defined as:

*Sub* means "less than"

*lux* means "light or energy"

*ation* refers to "a condition of"

Therefore *subluxation* can be interpreted as "a condition of less energy."

Metaphysically speaking, correcting subluxations is more than promoting better range of movement and relief of pain. A chiropractic adjustment is the *restoration of energy flow* that produces a healthier state. Even though there is disagreement regarding the same event—one mechanical and one holistic—both philosophies are working toward helping patients discover and experience improved health.

How doctors work is largely determined by how they

view their own bodies. There are many types of doctors—those that do or don't have a particular faith or spirituality, some who show their personalities, some who hide their personalities and want to be perceived as "professional," etc. The relationship you have with your doctor will be based on your ability to resonate with his or her character, philosophy on health, and your expectations of what a good doctor should do.

In actuality, these differences are wonderful. It is up to you to find a doctor who can be a partner in your healthcare—one whose personality, philosophy, and style resonate with your own.

Side note: I consider myself to be friendly and function in a relaxed manner. I tell jokes and sometimes my patients tell me jokes. I talk with them about their relationships, family, and career choices. I share my life experiences if I feel they are valuable to the specific needs of the patient. Even though my ways are sometimes unorthodox, I decided a long time ago that I was going to practice how I wanted and truly enjoy every moment so I could be a living example of what is possible.

Once in a while, I will call my young male patients "bro" or "dude," if I feel it will help me relate to them. I have also addressed female patients as "dear," "sweetheart," or "sweetie." Is this good or bad? Friendly or unprofessional? Obviously, the answer depends on your view. I take pride in the fact that I am approachable and easygoing.

Because of this aspect of my personality, a few patients and colleagues have labeled me as being unprofessional. However, I can only be myself—and that is all you can do, too. Every step you take, even for what you believe is the right intention, you will notice that some people support you and others will challenge you. Ultimately, it is not right or wrong, it simply is what it is.

I share this with you because I want you to know that you are *supposed* to be both supported and challenged. This realization is a major key to dissolving your inner conflicts, i.e., you will never please everyone all of the time.

Whenever someone asks me how to find a chiropractor, I tell them it is like hiring an employee. You interview five and you pick the one you feel will work best with you. You will know in short order whether the fit is right or not. One doctor simply can't be the right fit for everyone.

What about other health-care practitioners you might consider—acupuncturist, medical physician, physiotherapist, traditional Chinese medicine practitioner, etc.? With an infinite number of choices to help you deal with a particular ailment, who should you choose, and for what reasons?

Finding the answer can be frustrating, but it doesn't have to be. It only requires that you develop some level of awareness and take responsibility for your health.

One of my eighty-six-year-old patients told me that she has learned that she is responsible for healing and finding answers *herself* because "my body holds my soul, and that's a pretty big responsibility."

I was floored by her comment, because, in my limited perception of elderly patients, I oftentimes view them as being guilty of putting the responsibility for their health in the hands of doctors, and not themselves. I have had countless opportunities to help the elderly, who typically refuse to use my chiropractic services because their god-like family doctor told them not to.

The truth is that *everything* works! You heard me—everything. But, here's the key: a return to good health depends less on the healing art and more on the intention of the practitioner, as well as your relationship and trust in him or her.

I egotistically started my chiropractic career by negating

the medical model of health. I believed chiropractic was the answer to the world's problems. After seeing many patients thrive under my care, especially when other forms of therapy had been unsuccessful, I boasted that chiropractic was better. I even had patients from other chiropractors come to me and achieve better results. My conclusion? "I must be really awesome. I am the best!"

At the time, I worked in a multi-disciplinary, integrated health center with massage therapists and naturopaths. I believed I was the only one with the answers. Then, the lessons came hard. Every time I became cocky or elated with my success as a healer with a particular patient, I was faced with a humbling lesson: another patient would leave and get the success they were looking for with a few massages, some acupuncture, or physical therapy, or sometimes they were given medication that seemed to solve their problem. Some patients were turned off by my cocky attitude and went to another chiropractor.

After banging my head against the wall, and treating thousands of patients, I learned one valuable lesson: Healing comes from within. Healing comes from being tapped into an intangible source that is accessible to everyone. I am only one of many facilitators to healing. I don't have all of the answers. I may have been trained to ask important questions, but the answers are already within the patient.

Healing comes with having certainty about what I am doing as the healer and also from the certainty the patient has for me. Healing comes from being present with the patient, and the patient being present with me. Healing comes from being in a state of gratitude. It requires balanced interaction between the practitioner and the patient. This interaction can be administering a pill, a spinal adjustment, an exercise program, or an acupuncture needle; it can come with herbs and diet—or anything with the right intention. Even listening to patients talk about their problems and giving a hug can facilitate healing. I have even witnessed healing from simply laying hands on a patient.

When someone asks me, "Should I see a chiropractor, a massage therapist, or a physiotherapist for this problem?" my answer is always based on my experience. My filter of the universe as it relates to health and healing is through the lens of chiropractic adjustments; and I know with certainty that chiropractic enhances a person's ability to heal and maintain health.

My experience has taught me that patients benefit when the different healing arts work in unison, when the practitioners' egos are removed for the sake of improving the patients' quality of life. In fact, the different healing arts often complement each other.

One of my greatest awakenings occurred when I realized that when I chose to focus on an intention that I had certainty about and was incredibly good at (adjusting spinal misalignments), and worked in conjunction with the naturopaths and massage therapists instead of trying to do the work they were incredibly good at (diet and herbs and supplements, and soft tissue muscle techniques), patients always got better results.

As I develop into a more complete healer, I realize the importance of including other professionals on my patients' paths to healing. Patients can begin a chiropractic care and massage therapy plan and then, when beneficial, be referred to a naturopath to get their body chemistry analyzed and assessed, and/or introduced to a counselor or life coach to help with their emotional well-being and to help clearly define exactly what they want out of life.

Even if your spine is in perfect alignment, you can't express your full health potential if your diet is incongruent with your health goals. Have you seen otherwise healthy individuals suddenly "fall victim" to diseases? There is a reason: even if you are taking adequate care of your body with exercise, proper diet, regular massages, chiropractic adjustments, colonics, and vitamin supplementation, you could fall victim to an unbalanced emotional state and create diseases.

For overall good health, I suggest you use a complementary approach, do your research, and find practitioners that are right for you. To receive the most "wisdom for healing," address all of your needs: the structural component (muscular and skeletal/spinal system balance) with chiropractic, massage, acupuncture, and physical therapy; chemical component (vitamins, herbs, diet, various cleanses) with naturopathic care and colon hydrotherapy; and the spiritual/emotional component (meditation, counseling, researching, coaching, personal development seminars) with counselors and life coaches.

The quest for a healthy life is a journey. There is no solitary answer. In fact, it is ever-changing. Your results will accelerate if you have faith, confidence, and belief in the products, services, and ideas of the practitioners you choose—which is why it is critical to choose carefully.

You can tell within five minutes if the practitioner you are seeing is right for you. Do they like what they do? Would they rather be somewhere else? How confident are they in themselves and in what they do? Do they greet you with kindness and an enthusiastic attitude, or are they bullying? Are they rushed and inconsiderate? How do you feel about them?

Only you can be the judge.

## The Structural Component to Healing

Chiropractic college taught me to be a great human body

technician and to locate and correct the cause of many ailments. For example, headaches present with particular signs and symptoms, and chiropractors have the ability to locate the cause, which is often nerve impingement at the base of the skull or other areas in the neck. With a series of spinal corrections, called *adjustments*, signs and symptoms resolve and the patient achieves better health and well-being.

Chiropractic works. It gets amazing results, period.

I clearly remember a patient who presented to my office about one month after being in a motor vehicle accident. She complained of a massive headache that began immediately after the accident. Not one moment since, had she been without this pain. She had resorted to a daily dose of Tylenol-3; but still the headache made life unbearable.

Can you imagine what life must be like having a constant headache for more than thirty days? Can you imagine what her liver was going through to process and clear out the medication from her bloodstream?

This was her first visit ever to a chiropractor—her doctor had told her unequivocally, "DO NOT GO TO A CHIROPRACTOR." She came to me out of sheer desperation. Despite fearing for her life, she lay down on the exam table and I performed a thorough spinal examination.

After determining that there was obvious dysfunction that chiropractic could help, I reported my findings and she agreed to her first chiropractic adjustment. After this first adjustment to her neck, she got up from the table, dumbfounded, and said, "I can't feel my headache anymore!" Even though her symptoms improved immediately, correction of the dysfunction caused by the car accident was suggested.

Her treatment plan started with spinal corrective care (a series of adjustments synchronized with massage therapy and acupuncture over the next several months to stabilize and hold her corrections). In time, her adjustments started holding their corrections to the point where she only required maintenance care with home-based physical therapy.

Hers is one of millions of success stories that any chiropractor can share with you.

The most effective use of chiropractic care I have experienced in practice has been related to patients such as this lady, people who come in with physical symptoms that are clearly caused by physical stress—accidents, repetitive motion, falls, sports injuries, improper posture at work or rest, etc.

In her case, because the cause was a structural dysfunction, structural corrections with chiropractic (massage and acupuncture to speed up her recovery) helped balance her spine and improved her overall health.

Once the cause of a problem is identified by getting a case history from the patient, the examination allows chiropractors to locate the epicenter of the problem. From there, we can prescribe an adjustment style and corrective plan specific to each patient with great ease and success.

The motor vehicle accident victim in question received the benefits she was searching for. Her headaches disappeared and she also reduced her thyroid medication in half! It seems as a result of clearing the imbalances in her nerve system, her doctors noticed that her thyroid gland was functioning more effectively. She discovered that her thyroid levels were nearing normal and could only attribute this change to chiropractic care.

Yes, normalized nerve system function allows the body to work as it was designed to.

Although most patients spoke of their health successes under my care, I questioned why some patients got only temporary results or none at all. What about them? Why couldn't my adjustments solve their problems? This situation was very frustrating—but it was and continues to be the impetus for my continued professional growth.

## The Emotional Component to Healing

Stress comes from the inability to adapt to an ever-changing environment. Once I realized that the only thing in the universe I have the power to control is my thoughts, I decided that if I wanted to master my own life and not allow the roller coaster of highs and lows to take away my sanity, I needed to discover a way to balance my thoughts and emotions. Despite all my efforts to remove anything negative from my life, to avoid toxic people and forgive anyone who I perceived had wronged me or forgive myself for wronging others, I still experienced days of sorrow and despair.

I wanted to get away from living like those around me—in a constant state of panic and fear. I had to find a methodology to help dissolve inner and outer conflicts and, therefore, promote my own health and healing.

Research guided me to the work of Dr. John Demartini. After hearing him speak while in my first year of chiropractic school, I decided he would be one of the mentors I would study on my road to becoming successful. His style and manner of speaking resonated with me, plus he was both a chiropractor and a public speaker—two professions I was determined to fully master.

After I had been a chiropractor for three years, I attended "The Breakthrough Experience," a workshop presented by Dr. Demartini. From that point on, I began an accelerated road to personal transformation. My career took an entirely different path—one towards mastering my life and living my highest inspirations and aspirations by doing what I *love* to do rather than what I was *expected* to do by some outside authority.

Today, I not only get to facilitate the physical healing of individuals and work with a dedicated team of inspired healers with the same goal—I also have the tools to facilitate emotional healing.

Dr. Demartini teaches that the quality of your life is based entirely on the quality of the questions you ask yourself. Putting that concept in place has allowed me to enjoy the answers to some of life's toughest questions.

What if you took all the events that happened in your life and looked at them in a completely new way? Could you see each event in a way that is more empowering to you? Could you choose to break through your fears and guilt and transform your life from the one you are currently living to the one you want and deserve to live? Could this new way of thinking improve your physical and mental health?

Each one of those questions can be answered with a yes.

The first step toward taking control of your life is to start seeing things in a totally different light. The main hurdle to overcome is to understand that we live in a neutral universe, and in this universe every event is neutral—until someone with a judgment places a value on it. We label things good and bad, depending on our values.

For example: is snow good or bad? Well, if you are a snowboarder or a cross-country skier, you probably look at snowflakes and see beauty, grace, and fun times ahead. If you run a snow plow business on the side, you rejoice at the snowfall. But, what if you are a golfer or a gardener? Your value system is different, so your perception of snow is different.

In actuality, snow is just a form of precipitation and is neutral; it is beyond judgment—as is everything else. Car problems, marriage break-ups, work-related injuries, the death of a loved one, health issues, and even so-called traumas and abuses are neutral when looked at from a purely unconditional state in the quantum world. The emotions you have for any of these events result from placing a positive or negative value on them, and seeing them from one side.

I have had the opportunity to work with many people, some who have suffered a great deal and many who are depressed and fearful. And I have seen them dissolve relationship issues, family problems, and financial uncertainties simply by looking at their lives in a different way. Stress and emotional conflict come from looking at your life in a one-sided fashion. Only by awakening to the other side will you see an event for the truth that it is—a neutral, balanced state of presence that is a stepping stone to fulfilling your highest mission and purpose in life.

One of my clients valued the fulfillment and success of her four children and her relationship with them. One of the challenges she consulted me for was conflict with her husband, who was addicted to several substances. She wanted her husband to change, to be more productive financially and more involved with her life and the lives of their children. She was resentful that he ran the family business into the ground with his drinking. Her family and friends had told her to move on, that he was "no good," and "good for nothing." She told me that deep down inside, despite all his faults, she loved him and wanted to make things work; but she wished that he would change to be more helpful.

I asked her a disturbing question: "What are the benefits of his drinking?"

She responded, as most people who live stressful lives in the conditional world of judgment would, "There are no benefits!"

"Not true," I replied. "There is no event that doesn't have

both sides to it. I'm asking you to become aware of the benefits, to bring your mind to a state of balance with it, so you can become more present, rather than living in the past. What are the benefits?"

By the time I saw her next, she had written a list with pages and pages of benefits. The fact was, her husband's drinking gave their kids an impetus to find work (some of the kids had two or three jobs in addition to going to school). They were involved in community activities and had established a social network of support to balance the challenges at home. She also noted that while other kids were out partying and getting involved in things she would rather not have her kids be a part of, her kids were busy with youth programs, working, being productive, and becoming clear with their mission and purpose.

"Can you see that because of your husband's drinking, rather than in spite of it, the kids are on their road to fulfillment and your values regarding your children's fulfillment are being met?" I asked. She had not realized the benefits until then, and her perception about her husband shifted.

Over the next few weeks, she noticed a change in the interactions with her husband. By becoming more grateful for him as he was, more present with him rather than resenting the past, and seeing that he had unknowingly served her in getting her highest values met (children's success), he seemed to have changed. They spent more time together and were more unified. The truth is, though, he never changed—her perception of him did. He was the same all along—but people go where they are appreciated.

If you don't appreciate people for who they are—they will go somewhere else. And sometimes, all it takes is shifting your perception.

## My Greatest Infatuation, My Greatest Resentment

Anything that you do not view with a balanced perception can control you. If you do not see balance and instead see someone or something (including yourself!) with more positives than negatives, you tend to attract conflicts, problems, and humbling circumstances to bring you back to your truth—the neutral, present state of equilibrium and balance in the present moment.

Let me explain. When I bought my dream car, I was *infatuated* with it (saw more positives than negatives). Every time I became extremely polarized with the perception of my car being great, guess what happened? Scratches, dents, flat tires, fender benders, vandalism, even theft. In the span of one year, I had to make five claims to my insurance company—resulting in the astronomical increase of my comprehensive deductible . . . from $300 to $4,000.

I realize that even though I teach these principles now, I am not immune to these lessons: Everything is neutral and if you don't take control of your emotions and perceptions and balance them out, the universe will do it for you. Anything you see as only a positive will prevent you from being present, and will control you. Anything you have a balanced perspective on, you get to run.

Is there something that you were once infatuated with? Perhaps a relationship, a job, a car, an exciting adventure or a vacation? I invite you to conduct an experiment. Go back in your life and find something that once infatuated you. What happened as a result? If you are like me, and most other people, and you take an honest look at these events, you will see that your greatest infatuations became your greatest resentments.

This is not because you are a victim. It is simply because your perceptions were so imbalanced that the universe balanced them for you. The accident on the vacation, the tragedy at the height of your greatest celebration, post-partum depression, the difficulties after moving to an exciting new place—all are events designed to equilibrate your perceptions. To help balance yourself, choose to be aware of your thoughts and perceptions.

A helpful tip that I use: Whenever you label something as good, quickly run a list in your mind of its drawbacks. This will keep you from being infatuated by something and devaluing yourself for not having it. And, this practice will keep you balanced, grateful, and present.

Since I have started to inventory my thoughts and emotions and used this simple exercise, I have noticed a deeper sense of balance and control over my emotional states. I encourage you to do the same.

Have you ever resented something or someone so much that it took up time and space in your mind? Resentments run you as well. They keep you locked in the past and prevent you from expanding in the now and into the future.

Anything you are not grateful for controls you by affecting the decisions you make. You will have a tendency to avoid something if you perceive it will cause you pain. This is the opposite of empowerment and freedom. You can take control again by looking at things in a completely different way, i.e., what are the benefits of the event or person?

This is the most challenging mental exercise I have ever learned. Our beliefs in our perceptions are so powerful that sometimes we aren't willing to look at something in a new way. Believe it or not, it is sometimes easier to stay disempowered and in "victimhood" than to become responsible for the events that are happening in your life. Seeing things as only negative keeps you the victim and allows you to be the recipient of social and financial support from friends and family. But, if you truly can see the duality that exists in every area of life and in everything (nice and mean, good and bad, kind and cruel), you have infinite power at your disposal.

At a recent seminar, I took my greatest fear (losing my business and going bankrupt) and I ran through this exercise with the seminar attendees. I listed all the benefits of this fear that was running my life. I was able to see how free and magnificent my life could be if I didn't have all the financial and managerial responsibilities of owning my practice and (currently) two condo properties. I saw this great fear from another angle. I kept adding to the list until I saw that even if my worst case scenario came true, I would still have magnificence in my life. I was free.

This exercise, like any other, becomes easier with practice. I encourage you to master it, as it is one of the keys to opening your heart to the presence of the divine order that exists everywhere in the universe.

> "People who say they don't have time to take care of themselves will soon discover they're spending all their time being sick."
>
> Patricia Alexander

After I completed the exercise, I was rejuvenated. My shoulders relaxed and I was more at ease with my staff and patients. I wasn't run by my fear—it didn't matter anymore. I felt myself become more present with the day.

This freedom is accessible to you at any moment; you only have to open your eyes to another possibility. It exists outside of you and inside of you. By taking the time and asking yourself the right questions to open your heart to the possibility of the other side of an event, you will be able to see it for what it is, and not be governed by it.

The great discovery I had about the road to recovery is that healing is a journey in self-discovery. It is a path that is paved with challenges, obstacles, support, humility, joy, and pain. All experiences and events happen to assist you to realize your mission and purpose.

Hippocrates, credited with being the founder of modern medicine, was quoted as saying that it is important to care for the spine because it is the source of disease. Today, we understand this to be true because we have seen the intricate relationship between the human frame and the master system–the nervous system. Caring for the structure of this amazing human body, with the careful application of proper diet and nutritional supplements, is equally as important as balancing your emotions and turning your fears of the future and guilt of the past into grateful states of empowerment. That is a more complete form of healing—one that I have dedicated my life to understanding.

If you are interested in learning more about Dr. Nima Rahmany, and are looking for an engaging speaker for your next meeting on personal development, health and/or spiritual development, please contact www.DrNima.com.

It is our hope that this book inspires you to discover your true power to be healthy.

Health comes from within—and it is yours to discover. As health practitioners, we are here to assist you.

May you live a life filled with joy, success, health, and happiness.

Gilles A. Lamarche, BSc, DC, DAc